SEXUALITY & Long-Term Care

UNDERSTANDING AND SUPPORTING THE NEEDS OF OLDER ADULTS

by

Gayle Appel Doll, M.S., Ph.D.

Foreword by
Peggy Brick, M.Ed., CSE

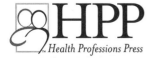

Baltimore • London • Sydney

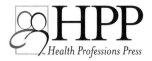

Health Professions Press, Inc.
Post Office Box 10624
Baltimore, Maryland 21285-0624

www.healthpropress.com

Cover design by Mindy Dunn.
Typeset by Barton Matheson Willse & Worthington, Baltimore, Maryland.
Manufactured in the United States of America by Sheridan Books, Ann Arbor, Michigan.

Information and suggestions provided in this book are opinions only and are in no way meant to substitute for the legal or medical advice of a qualified professional. Readers should consult a legal or health care expert for further advice or information and for applicable regulations, policies, or practices in their own state or jurisdiction. This book is sold without warranties of any kind, express or implied, and the publisher and author cannot accept liability for any resulting injury, damage, or loss to either person or property, whether direct or consequential and however it occurs.

Library of Congress Cataloging-in-Publication Data

Doll, Gayle Appel.
    Sexuality and long-term care : understanding and supporting the needs of older adults /
by Gayle Appel Doll.
        p.   cm.
    Includes bibliographical references and index.
    ISBN 978-1-932529-74-6 (pbk.)
    I. Title.   [DNLM: 1. Sexuality.   2. Aged.   3. Homes for the Aged.   4. Long-Term
Care.   5. Nursing Homes.   6. Sexual Behavior.   HQ 30]

    LC classification not assigned
    613'.0438—dc23
                                                                                    2011031138

British Library Cataloguing in Publication data are available from the British Library.

Contents

About the Author

Gayle Appel Doll, M.S., Ph.D., is Assistant Professor and Director of the Center on Aging in Kansas State University's College of Human Ecology, where she coordinates and develops research, educational and training programs, and outreach activities on aging. She received her Master's in Kinesiology and her doctorate in Life Span Human Development, both from Kansas State University. Dr. Doll teaches gerontology courses at Kansas State University, earning the Commerce Bank award for Outstanding Undergraduate teaching in 2005. Some of her courses are a part of the Great Plains IDEA distance Master's program in gerontology, an innovative online degree program managed through Kansas State University that incorporates professors of gerontology from six Midwest universities. Dr. Doll has also headed the PEAK-education team in developing educational materials to advance culture change in long-term care. Supported through the Kansas Department on Aging, the PEAK training modules were created to help long-term care staff to improve the quality of life for frail elders. One of these modules addresses sexuality and older adults. The background research for this work led to this book.

Dr. Doll's research has been published in *The Journal of Intergenerational Relationships* and *Activities, Adaptations and Aging*. In addition to her published research, she is active in community and state programs that promote successful aging and speaks extensively in state and national forums.

Acknowledgments

It would be impossible to try to thank all the people who have had a piece in this book. So much of my thinking about the subject of sexuality and aging has come from the many older lives that have touched mine. I've been comforted by the knowledge that our personality really doesn't change much over time. In terms of how this notion relates to this book—if you liked sex when you were young, you'll like it when you're older. I learned this from knowing some awesome people. I think of the Tuesday Ladies, older women I've met through my class and who have become great friends, and my own family members. But it's not just older women who have influenced me, but also women my age who give every indication that expressing themselves sexually is not going to go away when and if they decide to grow old.

There is a significant list of people who need specific thanks. At the top of that list are my dear friends and colleagues at the Kansas State University Center on Aging. Majka Jankowiak set the stage for this book with her pioneering work in research and development of training materials for sexuality in long-term care. Laci Cornelison helped put those materials into practice, and she and Majka field-tested many of the activities described in this book. Thanks to Pam Evans and Shelby Griffin for their technical assistance and cheerleading. My appreciation also goes to Migette Kaup, Stephanie Gfeller, Laci Cornelison, and Carol Marshall for their written contributions to the book. Thank you, Rick Scheidt, for giving me the confidence to share the knowledge that I have gathered from you and other great instructors I've known.

I'm grateful for Mary Magnus and Cecilia González at Health Professions Press for the assistance they have given to this rookie author to help complete this work.

My profound gratitude goes to the pioneers in the field of sexuality in aging adults, particularly Peggy Brick, who wrote the foreword for this book. They set the stage by getting people to openly discuss this once taboo subject. It is their untiring efforts that are helping to ensure that sexuality is seen as a basic human need, worthy of attention.

Thank you also to the long-term care providers and ombudsmen who shared their stories with me and to the older people who spoke freely about this subject.

Finally, thanks to my family. Mom and Dad, you showed me how hard work can result in seeing my dreams become reality. My kids may not know how much I love and appreciate them until their own kids have grown to adulthood, but Jake, Kemi, Caleb, and Jesse, being your mom has been an honor far beyond belief. Thanks for not only supporting me through this endeavor, but also for even bragging about me to your friends. If you can get me on *The Colbert Report,* more power to you. To Rick, I'll bet you never dreamed you were marrying a sex researcher 36 years ago. You've been there supporting me through every Gayle Doll re-invention. Thank you for your patience and your faith in me. You're the best.

Foreword

Sexuality and Long-Term Care: Understanding and Supporting the Needs of Older Adults is a vital addition to a growing movement protesting ageism and advancing the sexual rights of older adults. Although "humans are sexual from birth to death" has been the mantra of sexologists for many years, ageist stereotypes, reinforced by cultural traditions and media images, continue to portray people as non-sexual as they grow older. While earlier movements have targeted sexism, racism, and homophobia, only in recent years has ageism been identified as a major factor in how older adults are perceived and treated. Residents in long-term care, under constant surveillance and often diminished in both body and mind, are particularly vulnerable to having their sexual needs ignored, even forbidden. Gayle Doll's pioneering book not only integrates the growing research documenting the importance of respecting residents as full human beings, but also provides step-by-step guidelines for long-term care agencies that are ready to adopt a truly person-centered approach to validating and supporting resident sexuality.

Now, the word *sexuality* can be a problem. Many equate it with *sex* or *sexual intercourse*, behaviors associated with the young and not relevant to older adults in long-term care. Sexuality is, in fact, so much more! Sexuality includes one's feelings about oneself as a male or female person, body image, and the need for intimacy, touch, and connection. Acknowledgment of sexuality is a validation of one's whole self—a self not defined by the prejudices of administrators, staff, family, or other residents, or even of oneself. In *Sexuality and Long-Term Care,* Gayle Doll bravely addresses the many barriers—personal, organizational, social, and political—that currently deny the sexual needs and rights of many residents. I say bravely, because sexuality is controversial. Even supportive professionals will disagree with some of Doll's proposals. Great! Let us start talking, instead of suppressing, giggling about, or ignoring the sexuality of older adults.

Unfortunately, the only time many long-term care facilities address sexuality is when there is a "problem." Sexuality educators have known for years that sexuality education is generally deemed necessary when there is an increase in teen pregnancy, sexually transmitted infections, or sexual abuse. It was, in fact, a "problem" that first involved me in sexuality issues at the continuing care retirement community where I, joyfully, live. A widower moved in and soon developed a relationship with a resident with early dementia. It seemed a positive relationship for both; they ate together, held hands, and hugged. Some staff members, however, disapproved, particularly the younger staff. In-service workshops gave staff members the training and perspective for making important decisions about the woman's ability to consent. Only after the success of the workshops did the CCRC appoint an interdisciplinary team to develop the policy needed for responding to problems and for validating residents' sexuality.

Ideally, agencies should not wait for a problem to arise before they address the sexuality and intimacy needs of residents. Yet the day-to-day routines of staff and the medical demands of those in their care constantly trump the sexual and intimacy

Contents

About the Author

Gayle Appel Doll, M.S., Ph.D., is Assistant Professor and Director of the Center on Aging in Kansas State University's College of Human Ecology, where she coordinates and develops research, educational and training programs, and outreach activities on aging. She received her Master's in Kinesiology and her doctorate in Life Span Human Development, both from Kansas State University. Dr. Doll teaches gerontology courses at Kansas State University, earning the Commerce Bank award for Outstanding Undergraduate teaching in 2005. Some of her courses are a part of the Great Plains IDEA distance Master's program in gerontology, an innovative online degree program managed through Kansas State University that incorporates professors of gerontology from six Midwest universities. Dr. Doll has also headed the PEAK-education team in developing educational materials to advance culture change in long-term care. Supported through the Kansas Department on Aging, the PEAK training modules were created to help long-term care staff to improve the quality of life for frail elders. One of these modules addresses sexuality and older adults. The background research for this work led to this book.

Dr. Doll's research has been published in *The Journal of Intergenerational Relationships* and *Activities, Adaptations and Aging*. In addition to her published research, she is active in community and state programs that promote successful aging and speaks extensively in state and national forums.

needs of residents. Surely it will require a whole new understanding of the funda-mental importance of sexuality and aging before most long-term care homes are ready to dedicate their already pressured resources to creating and maintaining an environ-ment that supports the sexual health and wellness of its residents. And keep in mind that while this new understanding will be significant for current residents, the boomers are coming! Having already participated in the "sexual revolution," these newer arrivals will soon be insisting that their final homes acknowledge and support their sexual rights and needs.

In *Sexuality and Long-Term Care,* Gayle Doll recognizes the complexity of the issue and provides specific interventions for helping multiple stakeholders become supporters: administrators who are apprehensive about legal issues and family atti-tudes; professional staff who need knowledge and support; care staff who need educa-tion and clear guidelines; family members who are concerned about a parent's safety and dignity; residents who need acknowledgment of their sexuality without feeling shame and guilt; ombudsmen who need to be able to discriminate between abusive relationships and legitimate relationships.

The chapter case studies offer real-life scenarios that illustrate the importance of having an agency sexuality policy to help stakeholders understand and respond to sit-uations that arise. The scenarios are perfect for challenging people to respond to the classic sexuality education questions: How do you feel about this? What do you think? What will happen if . . . ? What could you do? In addition, the Activities following each chapter provide field-tested strategies that skilled facilitators can use to engage workshop participants in a variety of challenging situations. Professionals who wish to pursue Doll's recommendations but who feel anxious or embarrassed about dis-cussing sexuality and intimacy will find additional resources recommended through-out the book that can assist them, including The Sexuality and Aging Consortium, which I founded to address the fact that many agencies do not have staff who are ad-equately prepared to lead in-service workshops on sexuality and aging.

With *Sexuality and Long-Term Care,* Gayle Doll at Kansas State University's Center on Aging joins The Hebrew Home at Riverdale, New York, in seminal advocacy for the sexual rights of older adults. Since 2002, the Hebrew Home's video, *Freedom of Sexual Expression,* has been of inestimable value in advancing the cause of older adult sexuality. It shows administrators, social workers, nurses, and, perhaps most impor-tant, family members how to affirm the value of relationships between residents. There is, however, a paucity of resources supporting this movement. My favorite train-ing video, *The Heart Has No Wrinkles!,* is from Australia and is over 20 years old. (Both Australia and Canada have been far more active in validating older adult sexuality.)

I welcome Gayle Doll's contribution to the movement to confront ageism by understanding that older people are still people in need of love, intimacy, and recog-nition—that older people need to be seen as full human beings!

Peggy Brick, M.Ed., CSE
President, Sexuality and Aging Consortium at Widener University

Preface

Twenty, or even ten, years ago I never would have seen myself some day becoming a sex expert, especially not for the frail elder population. Now that I am starting to feel the part, it makes perfect sense.

A number of events occurred over the course of several years that significantly changed the way I view sexuality in older people. I was teaching an Introduction to Gerontology course in 2001, and, believing that it was important to expose my students to the "real deal," I was engaging older speakers for the class. I had heard about a group of women—the Tuesday Ladies—who had been spending one day a week together for 10 years. They would pick a spot on the map and trek there to try to discover something new and exciting. There were five of them, and they were all in their 70s. Their best trips were to bars in small Kansas towns where the local farmers would buy them beers.

I thought my students would love to hear their stories, so I invited the Tuesday Ladies to my house for brunch to convince them to speak with my class. Seated around the dining room table less than 10 minutes, they launched into a long and spicy review of their sex lives. I was a bit stunned. These women were a generation older than I, but they were having the same conversations I was having with my friends. Where was the generation gap? And, more important, what had I been thinking, assuming that sex would no longer be important to women of a certain age?

The second incident also occurred a few years later while I was teaching another gerontology course. I had started teaching classes at a local retirement community, which meant my "college-age" students were taking the class with 80-year-old men and women. During one class session I had to threaten to separate one intergenerational group of women because they could not stop giggling about sex—and that was not even the subject for the day!

The third event led to a great friendship. I was showing the film *Still Doing It* to the same intergenerational group. The film director interviewed nine older women about their intimate relationships (or lack thereof). The film is quite graphic in places, and when I showed it I chose to skip over a section that I feared would offend some of the elders. It turned out that the subject was far less uncomfortable for the older students than it was for the younger ones; one of the older women who wanted to see what I was afraid to show asked if she could borrow the film. I let her have it for a week, and she felt comfortable enough to invite her friends over for a viewing. I knew there was something special about this woman when she asked to borrow the film, and we have been great friends ever since.

I have studied many different aspects of nursing home care and have never been more intrigued with a subject area than I have with sexuality and older adults. Part of the lure has been that everyone else seems to be intrigued by it as well. While many nursing homes and long-term care organizations have not had formal discussions about resident sexuality and have not developed policies or staff training to address it, it is not hard to find people with plenty to say about it.

I am the director of the Kansas State University Center on Aging and my staff and I have conducted research to explore sexuality in long-term care settings. Much of what we have learned has been firsthand through interviews with nursing home personnel and ombudsmen, as there is a shortage of research on this subject. Most of the existing literature is from a problem focus, as if sexual expression in older adults cannot be viewed as normal or natural, especially when it occurs in a long-term care residence. Our initial endeavors were just to determine the need to explore sexuality in long-term care, and we were overwhelmed by the stories and the interest we discovered. Our research is presented throughout this book. You will find it in the stories told as well as in some of the statistics we have gathered.

When I told people the topic of the book I was writing (sexuality and older adults), many wondered if it was a subject that could fill a whole book, because surely most people when they get old could not care less about sexuality. If, however, we think about this subject critically, we learn that everyone is different and that, while some older adults may have no interest in sexual expression, others do. Instead, most of us think of sexuality in narrowly defined terms. While many older people are pursuing full and loving lives without engaging in sexual intercourse, most all of us need to be able to experience intimate relationships across the life span that are enhanced by a broad range of sexual expression.

The target audience for this book includes the persons most affected and most likely to react to and address resident sexuality—care staff, ombudsmen, and the state regulators who oversee long-term care facilities. The book also provides insights for administrative personnel as well as for family members.

It is my hope that this book will be used to guide discussions about beliefs and stigmas related to resident sexuality, provide ideas for staff sensitivity training, and encourage organizations to develop policies regarding resident sexuality. It is also my hope that by exploring resident sexuality readers will earn a greater understanding of each resident as a whole person.

Acknowledgments

It would be impossible to try to thank all the people who have had a piece in this book. So much of my thinking about the subject of sexuality and aging has come from the many older lives that have touched mine. I've been comforted by the knowledge that our personality really doesn't change much over time. In terms of how this notion relates to this book—if you liked sex when you were young, you'll like it when you're older. I learned this from knowing some awesome people. I think of the Tuesday Ladies, older women I've met through my class and who have become great friends, and my own family members. But it's not just older women who have influenced me, but also women my age who give every indication that expressing themselves sexually is not going to go away when and if they decide to grow old.

There is a significant list of people who need specific thanks. At the top of that list are my dear friends and colleagues at the Kansas State University Center on Aging. Majka Jankowiak set the stage for this book with her pioneering work in research and development of training materials for sexuality in long-term care. Laci Cornelison helped put those materials into practice, and she and Majka field-tested many of the activities described in this book. Thanks to Pam Evans and Shelby Griffin for their technical assistance and cheerleading. My appreciation also goes to Migette Kaup, Stephanie Gfeller, Laci Cornelison, and Carol Marshall for their written contributions to the book. Thank you, Rick Scheidt, for giving me the confidence to share the knowledge that I have gathered from you and other great instructors I've known.

I'm grateful for Mary Magnus and Cecilia González at Health Professions Press for the assistance they have given to this rookie author to help complete this work.

My profound gratitude goes to the pioneers in the field of sexuality in aging adults, particularly Peggy Brick, who wrote the foreword for this book. They set the stage by getting people to openly discuss this once taboo subject. It is their untiring efforts that are helping to ensure that sexuality is seen as a basic human need, worthy of attention.

Thank you also to the long-term care providers and ombudsmen who shared their stories with me and to the older people who spoke freely about this subject.

Finally, thanks to my family. Mom and Dad, you showed me how hard work can result in seeing my dreams become reality. My kids may not know how much I love and appreciate them until their own kids have grown to adulthood, but Jake, Kemi, Caleb, and Jesse, being your mom has been an honor far beyond belief. Thanks for not only supporting me through this endeavor, but also for even bragging about me to your friends. If you can get me on *The Colbert Report,* more power to you. To Rick, I'll bet you never dreamed you were marrying a sex researcher 36 years ago. You've been there supporting me through every Gayle Doll re-invention. Thank you for your patience and your faith in me. You're the best.

Foreword

Sexuality and Long-Term Care: Understanding and Supporting the Needs of Older Adults is a vital addition to a growing movement protesting ageism and advancing the sexual rights of older adults. Although "humans are sexual from birth to death" has been the mantra of sexologists for many years, ageist stereotypes, reinforced by cultural traditions and media images, continue to portray people as non-sexual as they grow older. While earlier movements have targeted sexism, racism, and homophobia, only in recent years has ageism been identified as a major factor in how older adults are perceived and treated. Residents in long-term care, under constant surveillance and often diminished in both body and mind, are particularly vulnerable to having their sexual needs ignored, even forbidden. Gayle Doll's pioneering book not only integrates the growing research documenting the importance of respecting residents as full human beings, but also provides step-by-step guidelines for long-term care agencies that are ready to adopt a truly person-centered approach to validating and supporting resident sexuality.

Now, the word *sexuality* can be a problem. Many equate it with *sex* or *sexual intercourse*, behaviors associated with the young and not relevant to older adults in long-term care. Sexuality is, in fact, so much more! Sexuality includes one's feelings about oneself as a male or female person, body image, and the need for intimacy, touch, and connection. Acknowledgment of sexuality is a validation of one's whole self—a self not defined by the prejudices of administrators, staff, family, or other residents, or even of oneself. In *Sexuality and Long-Term Care,* Gayle Doll bravely addresses the many barriers—personal, organizational, social, and political—that currently deny the sexual needs and rights of many residents. I say bravely, because sexuality is controversial. Even supportive professionals will disagree with some of Doll's proposals. Great! Let us start talking, instead of suppressing, giggling about, or ignoring the sexuality of older adults.

Unfortunately, the only time many long-term care facilities address sexuality is when there is a "problem." Sexuality educators have known for years that sexuality education is generally deemed necessary when there is an increase in teen pregnancy, sexually transmitted infections, or sexual abuse. It was, in fact, a "problem" that first involved me in sexuality issues at the continuing care retirement community where I, joyfully, live. A widower moved in and soon developed a relationship with a resident with early dementia. It seemed a positive relationship for both; they ate together, held hands, and hugged. Some staff members, however, disapproved, particularly the younger staff. In-service workshops gave staff members the training and perspective for making important decisions about the woman's ability to consent. Only after the success of the workshops did the CCRC appoint an interdisciplinary team to develop the policy needed for responding to problems and for validating residents' sexuality.

Ideally, agencies should not wait for a problem to arise before they address the sexuality and intimacy needs of residents. Yet the day-to-day routines of staff and the medical demands of those in their care constantly trump the sexual and intimacy

Introduction

*W*hat is *sexuality* and why is it so seldom spoken of when talking about older adults? The Sexuality Information and Education Council of the United States (SIECUS) has defined sexuality as a part of personality that encompasses sexual beliefs, attitudes, values, behavior, and knowledge. It is a significant part of who we are and what makes us unique. Because it is such an essential element of personality, it is important to help residents and staff in long-term care to deal effectively and compassionately with issues of sexuality. This requires a clear-eyed look at our own assumptions and possible misperceptions on the subject.

There are three domains that intersect and play a role in how people experience and express sexuality: biological, psychosocial/psychosexual, and cultural (Welch, 2011) (Figure 1.1). These three domains are constantly evolving, which also means that one's sexuality changes over the life span.

DEFINING THE COMPONENTS OF SEXUALITY

The biological domain relates to the inherited factors of maleness and femaleness, gender, and genetics as well as to how each contributes to sexual experiences. A few of the key issues associated with the biological domain are sexual differentiation (having to do with anatomical differences); sex hormones (which play key roles throughout life and certainly are important to the discussion of aging sexu-

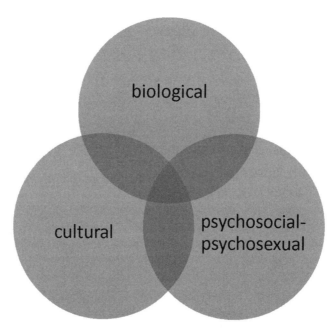

Figure 1.1   Sexuality domains

ality); sexual orientation (in this instance, the role of genetics, brain differentiation, and hormonal levels that contribute to orientation); and sexual health (freedom from disease, but also the role of physical and emotional well-being in sexuality). We, as a society, have made assumptions about the biological aspects of aging sexuality, including the belief that biological changes reduce or eliminate the ability or the desire to engage in sex and that without sexual activity people cannot be viewed as sexual beings.

The psychosocial/psychosexual domain of sexuality addresses psychological development within the context of social development and life experiences. Important elements of this domain include feelings and emotions, interpersonal relationships, and sexual health, which in this case refers to healthy attitudes and behaviors. The third domain of sexuality, cultural, relates to the influences that one's culture has on sexual attitudes and expressions, including the media, religion, and sex education. Chapter 2 discusses the three domains in more detail as they relate to aging sexuality.

Other Views on Sexuality

Sexuality may also be broadly defined as the quality or state of being sexual. It is a multidimensional concept that includes the desire for sex, beliefs about sex, and the sexual act. Many researchers have attempted to characterize sexuality. Here are some of their definitions:

- Hillman (2000) includes a combination of sexual behavior, emotional intimacy, sensual activity, and sexual identity. He further adds that sexual intimacy is the interpersonal relationship between two people who may or may not be engaging in sexual activity, placing an emphasis on the emotional experience and feelings of closeness. This definition works well with a life span perspective because many aging adults may substitute touch and closeness for intercourse as they grow older.

- Langer (2009) defines sexuality as the self-perception of being attractive as a sexual partner. The way a person dresses, speaks to others, and daydreams are all affected by sexuality and sexual identity.

- Kamel (2001) states that sexuality involves the whole experience of the person's sense of self, including the ability to form relationships with others, feelings about oneself, and the impacts of physiological changes as one ages on sexual functioning. (See Sidebar 1.1.)

Most people will immediately think of sexual intercourse when asked to define *sexuality*. The range of activities and behaviors associated with the term, however, can be quite broad and, in fact, for older persons, seldom involve activity between the sheets. Older people define and express their sexuality in more diffuse and varied ways than younger persons, which may suggest that changes in sexual expression and preferred sexual activity may commonly occur with advancing age.

Sidebar 1.1
Sexuality and Identity

Significant to the discussion of sexuality is its connection to identity. Females are most affected by this. Women are taught early in life to use their sexuality, that sexuality may be the most important aspect of the female identity. It can be used for "good" within the context of marriage or "bad" as in promiscuity. Sexuality for women is closely associated with youthful beauty and mothering young children. When older women lose their husbands or are no longer considered beautiful or needed for dependent children, they may feel depersonalized.

Understanding sexuality as multidimensional and not limited to sexual acts is an important first step in helping residents in long-term care to fulfill needs for intimacy and sexual desire.

INTIMACY VERSUS SEXUALITY

This book could easily have been about intimacy in long-term care rather than sexuality. While sexuality may better cover the range of activities and behaviors I present in this book, intimacy may be the story I'd rather tell. Miles and Parker (1999) wrote

> A major fear of the dying is that of loneliness, of dying alone. The barriers that the nursing home places to the development and nourishment of intimacy become profoundly important as residents near the end of their lives. As death approaches, it is too late to find or acquire the intimacy required to ease the transition and achieve a peaceful death. (p. 36)

Miles and Parker go on to define loneliness as the qualitative and quantitative deprivation of intimate relationships. A quarter of the persons living in nursing homes say they are lonely, with another 40% saying they are sometimes lonely. The solution to loneliness is relationships. Intimacy can be seen as a deeply rewarding and emotionally intense relationship in which someone can have another person with whom to share his or her dreams and feelings.

Another researcher, Judith Carboni (1990), elaborates on the loneliness concept by describing institutionalized elders as having feelings of homelessness that result from an overwhelming sense of loss of meaning of life. Residents mask their feelings by pretending to live in the past, surrendering to their circumstances, or distancing themselves from their situation and others around them. To alleviate this condition, we need to promote intimate relationships for residents. Intimacy or emotional closeness can act as a buffer in adaptation to stress and may be a requirement for survival as one grows older. The memory of being loved seems to continue to be important even for those whose cognitive abilities have diminished.

Langer (2009) emphasizes that one of the benefits of an intimate, caring relationship is increased self-esteem. She further asserts that love and sexual "turn-on" do not only occur in the purview of the young or beautiful. Langer, quoting Greer (1991), shares a lovely sentiment from the Lummis Indians of the Pacific Northwest who saw old age as the proper time to fall in love:

> It was the proper time to suffer romances, and jealousy and lose your head—old age, when you felt things more, and could spare the time to go dead nuts over a person, and understand how fine a thing it was. (Greer, 1991, p. 10)

Sidebar 1.2
Woody Allen

Woody Allen has stated that he will no longer play any romantic parts or cast other actors his age in any of his movies because, "Nobody wants to see a guy who's 74 hitting on a woman of any age." (As quoted in the November/December 2010 *AARP Magazine.*) European movies are more likely to show older lovers. Perhaps their viewing public is more conditioned to seeing romance between aging adults. Films such as *Something's Gotta Give* (2003) with older actors Jack Nicholson and Diane Keaton and *It's Complicated* (2009) with Meryl Streep, Alec Baldwin, and Steve Martin might suggest that American films may begin to follow the European lead.

All of us remember the first time we fell in love. Those memories do not fade easily, and the longing for a loving relationship does not diminish with age.

 Sexuality is the aspect of personality that supports intimacy and is greatly misunderstood, especially in older adults.

Sexuality is the aspect of personality that supports intimacy and is greatly misunderstood, especially in older adults. Most everyone can understand the need to develop intimate relationships. As Miles and Parker note, these relationships may become even more significant as residents struggle with end-of-life issues. By denying residents the ability to express their sexuality, we deny them opportunities to develop intimate, caring relationships.

To begin to think more openly about older adult sexuality, see Activity 1.1 and Sidebar 1.2.

TYPES OF SEXUAL EXPRESSION

Sexuality can mean many things, and for most older adults the range of sexual expression is much broader than for younger people. This means that older people feel comfortable expressing themselves in ways that do not always include sexual intercourse. In fact, in long-term care organizations the most frequent displays of sexuality involve flirtatious comments and women dressing up and having their hair and nails done to look attractive. These displays do not upset the normal routines

The goal should be to validate the sexual needs and desires of older people, not to make them feel pressure to be more sexual. We all have individual needs and personality differences. It is not appropriate to assume that everyone would be better off if he or she were involved in an intimate relationship. In fact, when one woman living in assisted living was asked to rate her sex life she said, "I haven't had sex since 1974 and that's just fine with me so I'd give it a 10!"

of institutional living. When sexual expressions go beyond those few that are seen as acceptable by staff, family, and other residents, however, problems often arise. Perhaps the first step toward alleviating these problems is to recognize that sexuality is an integral part of personality that does not vanish with age.

Sexuality can be expressed in many ways, including through words, gestures, or movements that may appear to be motivated by a need for sexual gratification. The desire to remain attractive, for example, is perhaps the most frequently observed display of sexuality among older women, with beauty salons reaping the benefits. The film *More than Skin Deep* highlights the importance that the beauty shop plays for older female residents. Few of us take into consideration that the weekly trip to have her hair done is the way that an older woman tries to express her sexuality—she wants to continue to feel attractive.

Kissing, fondling, masturbation, oral sex, and intercourse are also ways that many persons choose to express their sexual feelings. Other forms of sexual expression include touching, hugging, sending roses, providing comfort and warmth, dressing up, expressing joy, exploring spirituality, and maintaining beauty and physical appearance. Expressions of sexuality in nursing homes may include any of these examples, but more prevalently might be seen in flirtation and affection, passing compliments, and proximity and physical contact. Unfortunately, many expressions of sexuality are seen as inappropriate in nursing homes (see Chapters 4 and 6 for detailed discussions).

Perhaps one of the strongest tenets of aging is that as people grow older they become ever more diverse because of their histories as well as their health status. We should not lump all people together and we should not deny individual differences in sexual expression and desires.

DEFINITIONS OF TERMS USED IN THE BOOK

The following terms are used throughout the book and are to be understood as they are defined here:

Long-term care is used to describe the range of options for caregiving for older adults and may include home care, adult day services, assisted living, and nursing home care. While the primary audience for this book is nursing home staff, ombudsmen, and regulators, the material is also appropriate for those working in other forms of long-term care.

Assisted living is a type of care facility that is midway on the continuum of senior housing between independent living and nursing homes. These residences provide supervision and assistance with activities of daily living (ADLs).

> Perhaps one of the strongest tenets of aging is that as people grow older they become ever more diverse because of their histories as well as their health status. We should not lump all people together and we should not deny individual differences in sexual expression and desires.

Culture change identifies the process of changing the philosophy of a caregiving institution from a medical model to a person-centered model, addressing the holistic needs of residents, not just their medical needs.

Nursing home or *skilled care unit* is a residence that provides 24-hour supervision and medical services. Residents typically need help with a number of ADLs and have multiple chronic health conditions.

Ombudsmen are nursing home volunteers who advocate on behalf of the residents. Nursing home reforms introduced in the Omnibus Budget Reconciliation Act (OBRA) of 1987 and other congressional amendments related to nursing home regulations provide for the ombudsman as an advocate to help prevent abuse, neglect, and exploitation of older individuals in the nursing home setting. Ombudsmen serve as negotiators, problem solvers, educators, objective investigators, and collaborators who help facilities and residents achieve an equitable solution in situations that do not have clear solutions.

Person-centered care. This model of caregiving recognizes each resident as an individual with unique needs and desires and attempts to honor personhood through care provision that is directed by the resident's preferences. The goal of this model is the deinstitutionalization of long-term care residences, which includes honoring the caregiver as well as the person receiving care.

Intimacy. Intimacy refers to the feeling of being in a close personal relationship.

Sexuality. How people experience or express themselves as sexual beings.

GUIDE TO BOOK'S STRUCTURE

When sexuality, sexual expression, and sexual activity occur in the nursing home they can affect many people. This book aims to explore the perspectives of the resident, family, and caregivers. It provides educational opportunities for people who have not given this subject much thought and provides solutions and strategies for when sexual expression becomes a problem. These solutions may lead to common understandings.

Each chapter begins with a case study or story, all of them true and many from my own research on resident sexuality. These stories are meant to frame the discussion for the chapter, guiding the reader into making a personal connection with the content. They are also reviewed again at the end of the chapters for the purpose of discussion and reflection.

Key points are offered to emphasize important concepts. *Sidebars* illustrate information, many times by examining solutions that nursing homes or other long-term care settings have employed. *Activities* are offered throughout, and can be copied and used in groups or for personal reflection. A *For Further Information* list of additional resources on the content discussed in each chapter is included as an appendix to the book.

Chapter 2 presents residents' viewpoints. It provides research about what is currently known about older adult sexuality, sexual expression for older persons living in institutional environments, and the barriers to sexual expression. The chapter explains that while the cohort of adults currently living in long-term care has tended to suppress their sexuality, this may not be the case for future generations of residents.

Chapter 3 is about staff, including their biases regarding resident sexuality and suggestions for ways to address them. The chapter also discusses the benefits of successfully educating staff about resident sexuality and provides information about the components necessary for training.

Perhaps the most significant group to consider in a discussion of resident sexuality is family, the subject of Chapter 4. Guilt and confusion may cause family members to behave in ways that are upsetting to caregivers in the long-term care organization as well as to the residents. They may want to cling to memories of who their loved one was before the onset of dementia or frailty. This chapter helps staff and resident advocates to understand the emotions of family members and how to work with them to achieve the best outcomes for residents.

Over 50% of nursing home and assisted living residents experience some cognitive loss caused by some form of dementia (Alzheimer's Association, 2007). Sexual desire and expression exist for persons with dementia to varying degrees in the early stage of the disease. This can create myriad problems for staff because the long-term care institution is tasked with the responsibility of maintaining quality of life as well as protecting residents from harm. Staff can be faced with the dilemma of trying to determine the ability of a resident who has dementia to consent and make personal decisions regarding sexual expression. The affects of dementia on resident sexuality are covered in Chapter 5. Dementia may also lead to inappropriate behaviors, which is the subject of Chapter 6. Triggers for these behaviors as well as the solutions to address and prevent them are discussed.

An important aspect of sexuality is diversity. Many lesbians, gays, bisexuals, and transsexuals (LGBT) are expressing a fear that they will have to return to the closet and conceal their sexual identity because they believe that care providers will harbor biases against them or, even worse, may harm them. Chapter 7 discusses these concerns and presents strategies to train staff to exercise sensitivity when addressing the needs of the LGBT population.

The lack of privacy in long-term care is one of the primary barriers to resident sexual expression. The role of the environment is reviewed in Chapter 8. Much of this chapter was contributed by Migette Kaup, associate professor in Interior Design at Kansas State University. She consults with nursing homes in the development of environmental design that promotes positive outcomes for residents. This chapter also provides information about conjugal rooms.

Chapter 9 is a review of physical health issues that may provide barriers to human sexuality. It also covers safety concerns, as older adults are at high risk for sexually transmitted diseases.

Developing policy that addresses resident sexuality sends a message to residents, staff, and family that the organization considers sexuality to be an important aspect of the aging individual. Chapter 10 provides examples and meaningful activities that can guide any long-term care organization in the development of policies.

Finally, Chapter 11 offers a conclusion that is really more of a beginning.

Those who read this book will hopefully be much more comfortable in promoting healthy older adult sexuality and be prepared for what that may mean for their care communities.

REFERENCES

Carboni, J. (1990). Homelessness among the institutionalized elderly. *Journal of Gerontological Nursing, 16*(7), 32–37.

Greer, G. (1991). *The change: Women, aging and the menopause.* New York: Ballantine Books.

Hillman, J. (2000). *Clinical perspectives on elderly sexuality.* New York: Kluwer Academic/Plenum Publishers.

Kamel, H. K. (2001). Facing the challenges of sexual expression in the nursing home. *Long-Term Links, 11*(2), 1–6.

Langer, N. (2009). Late life love and intimacy. *Educational Gerontology, 35,* 752–764.

Miles, S. H. & Parker, K. (1999). Sexuality in the nursing home: Iatrogenic loneliness. *Generations, 23*(1), 36–43.

SIECUS Sexuality Information and Education Council of the United States (2009). Retrieved from http://www.siecus.org/index.cfm?fuseaction=Page.view Page&pageId=494&parent ID=472

Welch, K. (2011). *THINK Human Sexuality.* Boston: Allyn & Bacon.

Sexual Expression in the Media

Look for magazine pictures of older adults expressing their sexuality. How difficult was it to find an example? Compare it to pictures of younger persons displaying sexuality. What are the differences? Have you thought about the invisibility of older-adult sexuality? Can you think of any movies that featured older adults as lovers? Why are so many people uncomfortable with older people's sexuality? Think about how the sexuality we commonly see portrayed is from a problem focus (erectile dysfunction, low libido, senility).

Sexuality and Long-Term Care: Understanding and Supporting the Needs of Older Adults, by Gayle Appel Doll (Copyright 2012, by Health Professions Press, Inc.)

2

Sexuality and the Long-Term Care Resident

OBJECTIVES

- Examine older adult attitudes about sexual expression
- Illustrate the effects of ageism on attitudes about sexuality
- Assess personal beliefs about social norms
- Discuss actions that will enhance resident quality of life through intimate relationships and sexual expression

*A*lice had just moved to the assisted living home. She had not wanted to leave the little house where she had lived with her husband, John, for 56 years. After he died, however, her children feared for her safety because she had fallen several times. For the first 6 weeks she barely left her room at Golden Meadows, and staff considered having her assessed for depression. But then George moved in. He took an immediate interest in Alice and began courting her. The staff noticed a change in Alice— she was taking great care in her appearance and she was happy, spending more time in the public spaces, attending activities, and enjoying the meals with other residents. It seemed a win–win situation for all.

Peace in the home was soon disrupted when other residents began to complain about Alice and George holding hands in the dining room. The complaining residents, all women, thought that the occasional kiss shared by the couple was unseemly and should not be allowed. In addition, Alice's family questioned George's intentions with their mother. The staff worried that they may have to separate the two lovebirds to please the majority, knowing full well that doing so would negatively impact George's and Alice's quality of life.

It is very easy to state that all residents should be allowed to express themselves sexually. It is much more difficult, however, to try to balance this right to sexual expression with the rights of other co-residing elders who are simultaneously subjected to the behaviors.

A discussion about sexuality in long-term care must begin with an understanding of what older people need and desire. These needs should be examined from the perspective of the resident who expresses him- or herself sexually as well as from the viewpoint of the resident who may be the recipient of that behavior or others who may be subjected to viewing it on a daily basis.

OLDER ADULT VIEWS OF SEXUALITY

Until recently we have known little about older adult sexuality. Early studies suffered from methodological problems, such as few numbers of participants, lack of persons over the age of 60, and selection problems (much of the Kinsey Study was researched in gay bars). Within the last 10 to 15 years there have been a number of large surveys conducted for the purpose of gauging the amount of interest older persons have in sexuality (Sidebar 2.1). (An interesting feature noted by some of the researchers was that participants seemed to enjoy sharing information about this subject, refusing more questions about income than about sex.) A 2009 AARP study found that 45% of older men and 8% of women think of sex at least once a day (Fisher, 2010). Another study reported that most people between the ages of 57 and 85 think of sexuality as an important part of life (Lindau et al., 2007). The list in Table 2.1 is meant to establish the very clear message that older adults maintain an interest in sexuality throughout the life span.

Sidebar 2.1
If Life Had Been Different . . .

In one of my intergenerational classes (college students with older-adult mentors), I once asked, If people knew that they were going to live for 150 years would they live their life differently? Without hesitation an older woman in the front row raised her hand and blurted, "I'd have more lovers." "Georgia" was losing both her eyesight and her hearing and frequently complained of the many losses she had experienced, but her sexuality was foremost in her mind.

Table 2.1 Studies about older adult sexuality.

Study	Findings
Bretschneider & McCoy, 1988	Surveyed 200 older men and women: Frequency of masturbation and sexual intercourse does not change a lot after age 80. Touching and caressing without sex increases in importance, but may decrease in frequency after age 80.
Busse et al., 1985	Decline in sexual functioning seen with age but sexual activity and interest continue into old age.
Clements, 1996	*Parade Magazine* survey of 1,604 adults aged 65–97: 40% had sex an average of 2.5 times per month; 69% of men and 49% women reported that sex was important in their lives.
DeLamater & Sill, 2005	1,384 persons age 45 years and older reported that sexual desire decreases with chronological age, but that even at age 80 some expressed high desire.
Diokno, Brown, & Herzog, 1990	740 adults over the age of 60 were surveyed and reported: 73.8% of married men and 55.8% of married women continued to be sexually active. Among unmarried respondents: 31.3% of the males were sexually active and 5.3% of the women were sexually active.
Jacoby, 2005	AARP study with 1,400 respondents: (1) close ties with family and friends more important than sexual relationship to quality of life; (2) after age 50, the quality of the sexual relationship was related to the quality of the emotional relationship; (3) 30% of the men and 24% of the women between ages 60 and 70 had sexual relations at least once a week.
Lindau et al., 2007	3,005 adults aged 57–85 reported that sexual activity declined with age but 26% of 75-year-olds and above were still active.
Marsiglio & Donnelly, 1991	28% of 254 male community volunteers ages 66–71 reported having intercourse at least once a week.
Starr & Weiner, 1981	60% of men and 43% of women ages 80–91 remained sexually active.

In a very interesting paper, John DeLamater and Morgan Sill (2005) criticized the research on older adult sexuality, faulting it for reflecting primarily biological or medical perspectives on human sexuality. These viewpoints assume that as people age, hormonal changes, physical changes, or chronic illness reduce sexual desire and sexual behavior. These beliefs medicalize human sexual functioning and fail to take into account psychological and social influences on sexuality. Reflecting back on the domains shown in Figure 1.1 in the previous chapter, DeLamater and Sill agreed that the biological domain has been overemphasized for aging adults.

They elaborated on the multidimensional model, believing that older adult sexuality is influenced by the factors shown in Figure 2.1. Similar to the model in Chapter 1, Delameter and Sill proposed that the biological aspects include the hormonal and vascular systems as well as the effects of ill-

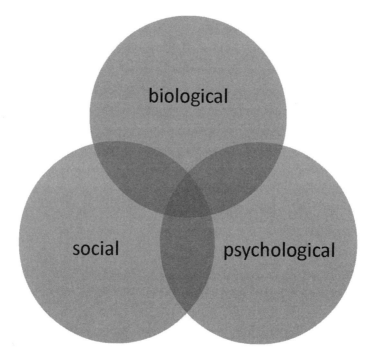

Figure 2.1 Sexuality domains redefined

ness and the treatment of illness. The differences between the two models is that the cultural aspect of sexuality has been dropped and the psychosocial aspects have been separated into two domains (social and psychological). The social influences identified by these researchers are clearly a departure from other work. They identified availability of a partner, the length and quality of relationships, and income. Psychological influences included sexual information, the attitudes that the older adult has about sexual expression, mental health, and the presence of depression or treatment of depression.

When Delameter and Sill applied their model to participants over the age of 45, they found that the major influences on strength of sexual desire for women were age, the importance of sex to the person, and the presence of a sexual partner. In men the primary motivators were age, importance of sex to the person, and education. Greater education is related to a more positive attitude about aging, which may undermine the negative stereotypes of older people and sexuality. This more positive attitude increases sexual desire. They also found that, overall, attitudes are more significant influences on sexual desire than biomedical factors. Because our attitudes about sex are socially constructed, a change in the societal view of the acceptability of older sexuality would be expected to increase the likelihood of sexual expression in long-term care. Because of the steady relaxing of attitudes about sexual expression in general over the past several decades, many experts see this pivotal change occurring in the not-so-distant future.

Sexual Desire

The literature is mixed on the motivation for sexuality. Early sex researchers saw sexual desire as a physiological drive or appetite that motivates the need for sexual behavior (Kaplan, 1977, 1979; von Krafft-Ebing, 1886/1965). Other researchers saw desire as an externally generated behavior; in other words, desire comes from wanting someone rather than arising from within the person (Velhust & Heiman, 1979). Still others would say that desire arises both externally and internally (DeLamater & Sill, 2005; Levine, 1987).

One finding that emerges from these studies is that desire seems to correlate with availability because many of the older adults who lacked partners expressed satisfaction with their sexual activity, or lack thereof. They seemed to feel that they were not missing anything. It has been suggested that older women who have been without a sexual partner for a long time drift into a state of sexual disinterest. "This is often a way of coping psychologically with their circumstances: by turning off their interest in something they don't have and see little likelihood of getting, they prevent themselves from becoming frustrated or depressed" (Masters, Johnson, & Kolodny, 1994, p. 479).

Widows often feel a moral obligation to remain faithful to their dead husband. Children who, consciously or unconsciously, may want this from their mom as well may encourage this feeling. Men may have similar feelings, but are more likely to remarry if their wife dies.

Cohort Influences

The beliefs of the cohort of older adults currently using long-term care have been strongly influenced by religion. When today's older adults were growing up their social life was centered in the church. The Judeo-Christian tradition of the early part of the 20th century in the United States encouraged prohibitions against sexuality, demanding repression of sexual thoughts and conduct. The church promoted virtue; it frowned on dancing, make-up, card playing, and other frivolity. Boys were told to "respect" girls, and girls were told that "good girls don't have babies." This tradition created a heavy burden of guilt and shame for some, specifically associated with nakedness, masturbation, and homosexuality.

Older people in the United States grew up during a period when sexual behavior was never discussed, sexual activity was suppressed rather than encouraged, and education about sexuality was minimal. Superstitions abounded, and many knew little about the facts of life. When women were pregnant, even when married, they were not supposed to be seen, and their condition was referred to as being "in the family way." Most parents did not discuss sex with their children, perhaps because they were not so very enlightened themselves. City-dwelling moms and dads purchased cats and dogs for the purpose of providing sex education. Farm kids certainly had exposure to copulation and birth, but whether they were able to relate that to human behavior is uncertain.

Modesty was an important value. Clothing was meant to cover the entire body. Showing too much leg was indecent and done only by fast or shameless women. Segregated swimming was normal, with swimming suits covering enough skin to make them drowning hazards. Menstruation left many women feeling ashamed and embarrassed.

It is significant to note gender differences in views about sexuality. Men have traditionally been more sexually active across all cohorts, except at 90 years old and beyond. Today's nursing home resident was influenced by conservative norms and double standards. Pleasurable sex was meant for men. Women were told that sex was for procreation and to please their husbands. Queen Victoria once told women to "lie back and think of England" in dealing with the sexual demands of their husbands (as their patriotic duty). This, coupled with the fact that there was no education about sex or sexual expression, left today's older cohort with very different ideas about sexuality than the generations that have followed.

> Several months ago I went to lunch with the Tuesday ladies mentioned in the preface. They are now in their early 80s. I told them about the book I was writing and asked them to tell me about what they knew about sex before they married. Most said they knew next to nothing, but one said that she was engaged to a boy who had had sex with a neighbor girl. When she had asked him what it was like, he had said, "Don't worry. Just 5 minutes and it will be over." This comment reinforced that sex was not believed to be a pleasurable experience for the woman—that she should just tolerate it for him.

Gender differences also persist in views about self-gratification. Masturbation is frequently seen more negatively in females. In a study completed in the early 1990s, 42% of men and 61% of women viewed masturbation in a negative light (Mulligan & Palguta, 1991). In the 1940s, 50s, and 60s, masturbation was seen as a sin, worthy of confession. Boys were told not to "waste their seed."

Many of the most persistent barriers to older adult sexuality are psychological in nature. Sexual attitudes, knowledge, and behaviors early in life are predictive of sexual desire. Younger people develop negative attitudes about older people and sexuality. The American culture values youth and reproduction, making sexuality inappropriate for those who are no longer young or fertile. Older people are told that they should be asexual, and when they are not, they are labeled as abnormal.

Attitudes Are Changing

If we were only thinking about care provision for the generation currently living in long-term care, we might be able to continue to avoid the subject of sexuality. Administrators and staff members could problem-solve as needed, and for most homes this would be a rare enough occasion that they could tolerate any of the behaviors that might arise. However, to be competitive, the long-term care industry must think ahead to the next generation that will inhabit these living environments—baby boomers.

Born between the years of 1946 and 1964, baby boomers came of age in a world that was more tolerant of sexuality. They reached adulthood when safe and effective forms of contraception were readily available, encouraging sexual activity for pleasure and self-expression rather than procreation alone. In addition, they had plenty of exposure to media that told them how to enjoy sex. This more open-minded attitude about sexuality, plus the sheer numbers of people in this cohort, suggest that the next generation moving into long-term care housing will be more sexually expressive. As evidence, there has been a disturbing rise in the incidence of HIV infection within this aging population. The cause is believed to be lack of condom use based on the reduced fear of pregnancy following menopause. (This issue will be covered in Chapter 9 on sexual health and safety.)

THE INFLUENCE OF AGEISM ON SEXUALITY

Ageism is a word coined by Robert Butler in 1987. Also called *age discrimination*, ageism is the stereotyping of and discrimination against individuals or groups because of their age. It happens all the time and everyone is guilty of it. Sometimes age discrimination targets young people, but more often it affects older adults. Here are some of the myths, or stereotypes, of aging: "You can't teach an old dog new tricks"; "Old people are useless, lonely, and depressed"; "Most older people live in nursing homes." Activities 2.1, 2.2, and 2.3 can be used with staff to identify and reflect on their beliefs or even stereotypes regarding aging, age norms, and older adult sexuality. It is important, for example, to explore further why people tend to think of older adults as asexual, because until we recognize that we are judging people and their actions based on deeply ingrained stereotypes, we will not be able to develop and implement new ideas and education to better address their needs regarding their sexuality.

WHAT WE KNOW ABOUT RESIDENTS AND SEXUALITY

The sexual attitudes of residents in long-term care mirror those of community-dwelling older persons—stated frankly, they want more than they are getting. While the desire for sexual intercourse does diminish, the need for intimate relationships and the need to be able to express oneself sexually do not.

Mulligan and Palguta (1991) interviewed 61 men in a veterans' home (average age 71) about their sexual attitudes and behaviors. Two-thirds of them expressed sexual desire but only a few were sexually active. Another study of 17 male and 23 female residents (all cognitively intact) found that sexual activity was infrequent among all (Spector & Fremeth, 1996). Men expressed higher levels of sexual desire than women and less sexual satisfaction. A much larger Texas study with 250 nursing home residents also found little activity (8% had been sexually active in the previous month), but significantly more residents (17%) reported a desire to be active (White, 1982). Finally, 63 nursing home residents in a 1979 study found that nearly all admitted to having sexual thoughts (Wasow & Loeb, 1979). The common finding across all of these studies is that libido persists even in frail nursing home residents.

The types of expressiveness most evident in residential dwellings may include flirtation embellished with humor and witty remarks. These types of communications frequently lead to affection. Residents can be observed passing compliments to each other about what they are wearing. People living in long-term care may show affection through proximity (sitting next to another person) and physical contact (the touch of a hand, a kiss on the check). Romantic behavior—holding hands, stroking, calling someone "special friend" or some other term of endearment—have also been observed (Sidebar 2.2).

BENEFITS OF RESIDENT SEXUALITY

The following is a list of benefits of resident sexuality that caregivers and researchers have observed:

- Pleasure
- Release of tension
- Communication

Sidebar 2.2
Kansas State University Center on Aging Survey Findings

In 2009 researchers at the Center on Aging at Kansas State University surveyed nursing home administrators in Kansas to find out how often sexual expression was demonstrated in nursing homes (Doll, Bolender, & Hoffman, 2011). Nearly all of the 90 administrators responding expressed that some activity was occurring on a relatively frequent basis. The chart below shows the frequencies of five types of sexual expression. Of course, there are many more, but the ones listed have been known to cause "problems" within the nursing home environment.

Figure 2.2   Types of sexual expression in Kansas nursing homes

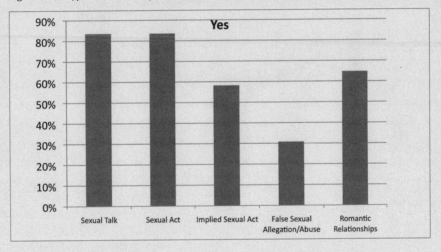

- Mutual tenderness
- Passion
- Affirmation of one's body and its functioning
- Sense of identity
- Security when the outside world is troubling
- Greater locus of control
- Increased self-esteem

A 2009 AARP study found that 45% of older men and 8% of women think of sex at least once a day (Fisher, 2010). Another study reported that most people between the ages of 57 and 85 think of sexuality as an important part of life (Lindau et al., 2007).

Bill Thomas (1996), one of the leaders in the culture change movement, believes that the three greatest problems in nursing homes are boredom, loneliness, and helplessness. He has suggested "curing" these problems with, among other things, the development of relationships that include intergenerational associations with children and the inclusion of pets in the facility. It takes very little imagination to see, based on the list above, that expressions of sexuality that may lead to intimate relationships would also be very beneficial to residents.

BARRIERS TO RESIDENT SEXUALITY

When people grow old in a culture that reinforces stereotypes, misconceptions, and humor about older adult sexuality, their own attitudes about sexual expression can be negatively influenced. Older men may compare themselves to younger men, thereby believing that they cannot live up to performance standards. On the other hand, they benefit from a societal belief that older men are handsome and distinguished, whereas women come to believe that only the young can be attractive.

The belief that sexual activity is socially unacceptable and possibly even physically harmful may have negative consequences for older adults. Fearing criticism and perhaps even laughter, older individuals may withdraw from all forms of sexual expression when it can still be beneficial to themselves and to their potential partners.

Adult children can contribute to the problem when they are reluctant to let go of their perceptions of parents in their roles as Mom and Dad. Adult children's attitudes toward their parent's sexuality may have a greater effect than disability or illness.

Likewise, the attitudes of staff members can be a deterrent to sexual expression. Biases about older adult sexual expression can perpetuate the feelings of guilt and inadequacy in residents who think that their sexual desires are abnormal. One study found that care staff were more accepting of sexual expression in people with disabilities, mental illness, and cognitive impairment than in older adults (Kaas, 1978). Another study found that, while staff members recognized older adults as having sexual desires and needs, they did not see the importance of offering support for those needs (Wasow & Loeb, 1975). The study revealed that staff used regulations, schedules, and treatments as excuses to avoid helping residents fulfill sexual needs. Judgments about what constitutes dignified behavior in older persons also contributed to staff not helping residents fulfill their needs.

Perhaps the most profound barrier for sexual expression in older residents is the lack of a partner. This is especially true for women, who are more likely than men to be widowed, divorced, separated, or single as they grow older. Men tend to die younger or move on to a younger woman. There are close to three women for every man in nursing homes, but because 75% of those men are married, the ratio of single or available women to men may exceed 4:1. Many researchers have reported that women do not choose to have sex outside of marriage, but marital status makes little difference to men. In the future we may see more unconventional relationships, as illustrated in Sidebar 2.3.

Lack of a partner is not a limit to fantasy, self-gratification, or masturbation; however, these forms of sexual expression are not real possibilities for people concerned about guilt, the lack of privacy, and the fear of being caught. Few private spaces exist in nursing homes, which were designed to allow for easy observation. Doors are left open and rooms are shared, separated only by draw curtains. Caregivers focus on efficient delivery of care and typically think it is acceptable to compromise resident privacy in the name of good physical care.

Resident sexuality and privacy are compromised in other ways. The option to have sex is sometimes controlled by the schedules and routines of the nursing home. If sexual activity is condoned in a home, it may only be allowed between bathing, meals, nap times, and other regimented activities.

Sidebar 2.3
Maggie Kuhn

Maggie Kuhn, the founder of the Gray Panthers, once got herself into trouble by suggesting to a group of women at a church conference that if they found themselves in the position of not having a partner late in life, they should consider becoming lesbians. Her suggestion may have made a lot of practical sense as a tactic for avoiding loneliness, but Kuhn may have been a bit before her time. As people become more accepting of a wider range of sexual expression we may see more women choose to develop intimate relationships with other women to avoid the isolation of nearing death alone.

Another barrier to resident sexuality is the problem of maintaining the privacy of patient information. Behaviors that impact the care of the resident must be documented. Many residents may abstain from sexual activity to avoid having it be documented and possibly become public knowledge or the subject of gossip.

The residents themselves may be another barrier to resident sexual expression. Older people have been socialized to carry deeply ingrained notions about what is right or unseemly for people of their age. They may disapprove of sexual expression in their fellow residents. Not uncommon is the disapproval that comes from jealousy. For some, if *they* cannot have a relationship, then no one else should either. Completing Activity 2.4 will help you to identify the types of barriers to sexual expression that may exist in your facility.

It has been speculated that residents in long-term care settings have a greater need for sexual intimacy than other older persons because of the cumulative losses of functional ability, a spouse, finances, social roles, and the like. When these losses are experienced, an emotional closeness to someone may rebuild the resident's self-esteem. When residents feel good about themselves, they feel better about other residents as well as staff.

STRATEGIES FOR MEETING RESIDENT SEXUALITY NEEDS

Many persons who work with older adults in care facilities may not be aware that there are several ways to fulfill a resident's needs regarding sexuality and intimacy. It can be as simple as learning to touch the resident appropriately or a facility may decide to provide a room for conjugal visits (see Chapter 8). Most strategies involve the development of meaningful relationships and are described in the sections that follow.

Touch

The need for human touch is universal throughout the life span. Touch is a way of demonstrating intimacy. A lack of intimacy can inhibit mental health, development, and maturity. The way a person is touched can be a delicate balance between providing intimacy or overstepping and being intrusive.

In caregiving, touch can be either task- or nontask-related. Task-related touch includes taking a pulse, bathing, grooming, or applying a bandage. Nontask-related touch may include hugging, patting a hand, or stroking a cheek. This kind of touching is expressive or nonverbal communication. Touch is important for the resident's sense of identity and self-esteem. In one study a correlation was found between light touching and improved appetite in persons with dementia (Ostuni & Pietro, 2001).

It is important to appreciate that touch can be perceived differently by different residents. Some may find it comforting and important, while others find it aversive. The reactions may be cultural in origin or based on the resident's history. Some residents may be unfamiliar with being touched and may misinterpret it as a sexual advance. Caregivers should be sensitive to individual differences and use touch appropriately. The caregiver's own attitude about touching may have a lot to do with how residents react to skin contact. One study found that 70% of care providers felt ill at ease about touching older residents (Huss, 1977). These attitudes are unconsciously passed on to the resident. According to Hollinger and Buschmann, residents perceive touch positively if the following three conditions are met: (1) touching is perceived as adequate for a given situation; (2) no greater intimacy is forced on the resident than he or she desires; (3) caregivers do not use a condescending attitude (Hollinger & Buschmann, 1993).

Much of the care provided to older adults in institutions is intimate care because it must involve invading the care receiver's privacy. Given this fact, care should be delivered under the resident's terms. Caregivers should try to determine the level of touch and manner of speaking that makes the resident feel most comfortable.

> I once observed a caregiver who was providing intimate care for a person with ALS (amyotrophic lateral sclerosis—Lou Gehrig's disease). So that he could maintain as much control as possible, she asked his permission for everything she did for him. "Now, is it OK if I move this leg just a little? Would you like to have a sip of water? It's time for your exercises. Which one would you like to do first?" I left that day having learned a tremendous lesson about human dignity.

The following list includes ways to incorporate touch into caregiving activities:

- *Hair grooming.* Doing hair serves several purposes. It promotes touch, feels good, and enhances self-esteem through perceived improvements in attractiveness.
- *Hand massage.* The addition of aromatic lotions seems to have therapeutic effects. An ideal time to engage in this activity is while residents are waiting for a meal or an activity to begin. Be aware of residents who may have painful arthritis and may not enjoy this activity.

- *Manicures and pedicures.* Many women take pride in their hands. This activity is especially good because it promotes face-to-face conversations.

- *Range of motion exercises.* This is an ideal time for meaningful conversation.

> When one of my sons was young he wanted to pass the President's Challenge on physical fitness at his grade school, and asked for my help with his flexibility. As I helped him with stretches I got to touch him a lot at a time in his life when it was not "cool" to be associated with Mom. We had great conversations, and he won the award!

- *Taking the resident's pulse.* For staff who may be uncomfortable with touching, there are plenty of ways to incorporate it into normal routines. When providing a clinical checkup such as blood pressure and pulse measurements, just add some comments about the resident's dress or new shirt and you've done your job.

- *Back rubs.* Bodies get achy with too much sitting. You can help with a quick rub and a pat.

Keep in mind that it is important to know the resident. Some may not desire any touch at all. Some will need to build trust in you before they accept it. Be respectful of each resident's desires and tolerances.

Consistent Staffing

One of the hallmarks of person-centered care is consistent staffing and assignment. This means that the same caregivers are consistently assigned to the same set of residents. The caregiver and the resident get to know each other well, increasing the likelihood of a close and caring relationship. Quality of life can improve when residents know someone understands and accepts them. When residents are taken care of by the same person as much as possible, they report higher perceptions of choice and control.

Research has documented other benefits for residents when staff members are consistently assigned to the same residents, including a reduction in the incidence of pressure ulcers, a decrease in the rate of patient death, and an increase in the number of ambulatory residents (Campbell, 1985). Consistent staffing has also been shown to improve continence for older residents; when caregivers know the residents, they learn their personal habits and can take them to the bathroom prior to an accident (PEAK, 2006). Consistent staffing also improves family satisfaction as the family members and staff form relationships (Farrell & Frank, 2007).

On a larger scale, long-term care organizations benefit from permanent assignment because caregiver turnover rates have been shown to decline (Farrell & Frank, 2007). Caregivers plan to stay because they feel valued, and those who are permanently assigned feel a higher sense of accountability.

Less well known to the residents are their nighttime and weekend caregivers.

In one facility, each staff member was appointed a "care advocate" for one resident. The advocates were responsible for getting their resident to and from appointments and communicating with the family about needs and care plan meetings. The purpose of this commitment was to increase the development of close personal relationships. Staff confirmed that it helped them to forge intimate relationships not only with the resident, but also with the resident's family.

Frequently these staff members are not consistently assigned, and it is in these periods of the day when problems may arise. Activity 2.5 describes methods to help staff understand the benefits of consistent assignments.

Counseling and Education

Residents should be provided with education and counseling, if desired. In a facility where the sexuality policy is open and easily accessible, residents and family members will be more likely to express interest. There may also be a need for medical support for some sexual activities. Condoms, performance-enhancing drugs, and vaginal lubricants should be available. Residents can be counseled about other forms of sexual gratification outside of intercourse. Education should include the risk of sexually transmitted disease. A positive relationship exists between knowledge and attitudes toward sexuality in later life. With education, residents can both feel better about expressing their own sexuality and be more understanding of that expression in other residents.

Because of the general asexual culture of the nursing home, some residents may think they are abnormal if they have sexual feelings. Good videos are available to help staff, families, and residents understand and accept that sexual feelings can endure through a lifetime. *Back Seat Bingo* is a 6-minute video in which older adults describe their needs for intimacy. *Still Doing It* follows nine aging women who describe how they gratify their own sexuality. Open discussions among staff and residents following these viewings will allow people to express their own feelings.

DISCUSSION

Return to the story of Alice and George that begins the chapter. How could the facility staff manage the situation? How is their relationship similar to or different from new relationships at other ages? What could this facility or others do to avoid future problems such as this?

SUMMARY

Ageist beliefs have created a culture in which older adults are expected to be asexual. Older adults themselves may suppress sexual feelings as they find themselves lacking in opportunities to fulfill their needs and also as they try to conform to societal beliefs and mores.

Older adults living in long-term care facilities, however, may have an even greater need for sexuality and intimate relationships than their counterparts living in the community. Institutional living can strip a person of freedom and control, leaving a tremendous sense of loss. Sexuality can be a positive experience when faced with these losses and the inevitability of death.

Staff and family members need to examine their own ageist beliefs if they are to be successful in helping the older adult resident fulfill basic needs and desires and improve the quality of life in long-term care.

REFERENCES

Bretschneider, J. G., & McCoy, N.L. (1988). Sexual interest and behavior in healthy 80 to 102-year-olds. *Archives of Sexual Behavior, 17*(2), 109–129.

Busse, E. W., Maddox, G. L., Buckley, C. E., Burger, P.C., George, L. K., Marsh, G. R., et al. (1985). *The Duke longitudinal studies of normal aging: 1955–1980.* New York: Springer.

Butler, R., & Lewis, M. (1987). Myths and realities of sex in later years. *Provider, 13,* 11–13.

Campbell, S. (1985). Primary nursing: It works in long-term care. *Journal of Gerontological Nursing, 8,* 12–16.

Clements, M. (1996). Sex after 65. *Parade Magazine. 4–5. 7.*

DeLamater, J., & Sill, M. (2005). Sexual desire in later life. *Journal of Sex Research, 42*(2), 138–149.

Diokno, A. C., Brown, M.B., & Herzog, A. R. (1990). Sexual function in the elderly. *Archives of Internal Medicine, 150,* 197–200.

Doll, G., Bolender, B., & Hoffman, H. (2011). Sexuality in nursing homes: Practice and policy. Manuscript submitted for publication.

Farrel, D. & Frank, B. (2007). A keystone for excellence, *Provider, 33*(7), 35–37.

Fisher, L. (2010). *Sex, romance and relationships: AARP survey of midlife and older adults.* Washington, DC: AARP.

Hollinger, L. M., & Buschmann, M. (1993). Factors influencing the perception of touch by elderly nursing home residents and their health caregivers. *International Journal of Nursing Studies, 30,* 445–461.

Huss, A. (1977). Touch with care or caring touch? *American Journal of Occupational Therapy, 31,* 11–18.

Jacoby, S. (2005). Sex in America. *AARP Magazine.* Retrieved from http://www.aarpmagazine. org/lifestyle/relationships/sex_in_america.html

Kaas, M. (1978). Sexual expression of the elderly in nursing homes. *The Gerontologist, 18*(4), 372–378.

Kaplan, H. (1977). Hypoactive sexual desire. *Journal of Sex and Marital Therapy, 3,* 3–9.

Kaplan, H. (1979). *Disorders of sexual desire and other new concepts and techniques in sex therapy.* New York: Brunner/Mazel.

Levin, S. (1987). More on the nature of sexual desire. *Journal of Sex and Marital Therapy, 13,* 35–44.

Lindau, S. T., Schumm, L. P., Laumann, E. O., Levinson, W. L., O'Muircheartaigh, C., & Waite, L. J. (2007). A study of sexuality and health among older adults in the United States. *New England Journal of Medicine, 357*(8), 762–774.

Marsiglio, W., & Donnelly, D. (1991). Sexual relations in later life: A national study of married persons. *Journal of Gerontology, 46*(6), S338–S344.

Masters, W., Johnson, V., & Kolodny, R. (1994). *Heterosexuality.* New York: Harper Collins.

Mulligan, T., Palguta, R. F. (1991). Sexual interest, activity, and satisfaction among male nursing home residents. *Archives of Sexual Behavior, 20,* 199–204.

Ostuni, E., & Pietro, M. J. (2001). Effects of healing touch on nursing home residents in later stages of Alzheimer's disease. (Abstract). Healing Touch International, 5th Annual Conference, Denver, CO.

Pallmore, E. (1998). *The facts on aging quiz,* 2nd ed. New York: Springer.

PEAK (2006). Sexuality in long-term care. *Promoting Excellent Alternatives in Kansas Nursing Homes.* Retrieved from http:www.agingkansas.org/LongTermCare/PEAK/peak.htm# modules.

Spector, I. P., & Fremeth, S. M. (1996). Sexual behavior and attitudes of geriatric residents in long-term care facilities. *Journal of Sexual Marital Therapy, 22,* 235–246.

Starr, B. D., & Weiner, M. B. (1981). *The Starr-Weiner report on sex and sexuality in the mature years.* New York: Stein & Day.

Thomas, W. (1996). *Life worth living: How someone you love can still enjoy life in a nursing home: The Eden Alternative in action.* St. Louis: Vanderwyk and Burnham.

Velhust, J., & Heiman, J. (1979). An interactional approach to sexual dysfunctions. *American Journal of Family Therapy, 7,* 19–35.

von Krafft-Ebing, R. (1886/1965). *Psychopathia sexualis.* New York: Putnam.

Wasow, M., & Loeb, M. B. (1979). Sexuality in nursing homes. *Journal of the American Geriatric Society, 27,* 73–79.

White, C. B. (1982). Sexual interest, attitudes, knowledge, and sexual history in relation to sexual behavior in the institutionalized aged. *Archives of Sexual Behavior, 11,* 11–21.

An Aging Stereotype Quiz

To test your beliefs regarding aging, answer *true* or *false* to the following questions.

1. ____True   ____False   The majority (more than 50%) of older adults will become senile (memory loss, disorientation, dementia) during old age.

2. ____True   ____False   Most older adults have no desire or capacity for sexual relations. In other words, most older adults are typically asexual.

3. ____True   ____False   Chronological age is the most important determinant of someone's age.

4. ____True   ____False   Declines in all five senses normally occur at old age.

5. ____True   ____False   Intelligence tends to decline at old age.

6. ____True   ____False   In general, most older adults tend to be pretty much alike.

7. ____True   ____False   The majority of older adults say that they are lonely.

8. ____True   ____False   Old age can be characterized as a second childhood.

(See the answers to this quiz at the end of the chapter.)

Source: Based on Palmore's work with stereotypes (1998). Adapted from Aging Quiz, Linda M. Woolf, Webster University at www.webster.edu/~wolflm/myth.html. Be sure to check the website for additional questions.

Answers to Aging Stereotype Quiz (Activity 2.1)

1. *False.* The majority of older adults do not become senile. Dementia is not a normal part of aging. It is only after the age of 85 that as much as 50% of the population may have some form of dementia. The numbers are far lower at earlier ages.

2. *False.* Sexuality continues to be an important part of the older adult's life. People can enjoy sexual relationships well into late life. Sexuality need not be considered as merely a biological function. Sexual expression can take many forms.

3. *False.* People age in many different ways, and chronological age is the least important. It is more important to consider functional age, which is made up of psychological age, social age, and biological age. Everyone is different.

4. *True.* Most people will experience some declines in the five senses as they age.

5. *False.* For the most part, any declines in intellectual functioning may be caused by disease rather than age.

6. *False.* Older adults are more diverse than any other age population, as they have had years of varied experiences and developmental opportunities.

7. *False.* Although loneliness is one of the greatest fears of older people, two-thirds report rarely, if ever, feeling lonely.

8. *False.* Older adults are adults and always should be treated as such, even if incapacitated because of disease.

Age Norms

Even caregivers who believe themselves to have an affinity for older adults can harbor ageist beliefs, especially when it comes to expressions of sexuality. Part of this is because we are socialized to associate an appropriate age to certain activities. Read through the following list and think about the age for which each is generally associated. If you are old enough to remember 20–30 years ago, think about how these norms may have changed over time.

What age is most commonly associated with the following?

Marriage _____	Graduating from high school _____
First drink _____	Driver's license _____
Grandparenthood _____	First vote _____
College _____	Graduate school _____
Having children _____	Tattoos _____
Rap music _____	Cover model _____
Medicare _____	AARP _____
Condoms _____	Hot sex _____

As you read through this list it may occur to you that most of these age norms have become far more variable or flexible over the years. The average age of first marriage has gone up consistently and is currently 27.7 for males and 26 for females, but the national average age of first pregnancy has not changed much because of large numbers of teen pregnancies. AARP used to be for "retired" persons, but now they heavily advertise for the just-turned-50 crowd. Members of this group are also reinventing themselves by going back to school or getting a tattoo to commemorate life changes.

The point of this activity is to help participants understand that assigning appropriate ages for activities is a fruitless and meaningless endeavor. People have the right to do what seems best for them at the time that they deem is right, and that includes having intimate relationships long past the age that has been accepted by society.

Sexuality and Long-Term Care: Understanding and Supporting the Needs of Older Adults, by Gayle Appel Doll
(Copyright 2012, by Health Professions Press, Inc.)

Birthday Cards and Ageism

Collect birthday and anniversary cards, jokes related to aging, and magazine ads that highlight sexuality. Using these types of materials to educate staff about ageist beliefs can be very effective. Have staff review these materials and discuss the facts to support or refute the assumptions made by each. For example, a cartoon may derive its humor from implying that an older couple has just experienced a satisfying sexual experience. Because we make assumptions that all older people are asexual we exclude all noncoital forms of sexual expression as sexually satisfying for older adults and as improving quality of life. The reality for many older adults is that the desire for sexual intercourse may be replaced by a need for intimacy that can be expressed by cuddling, holding, caressing, and other noncoital activities.

Use the cards to discuss the ageism apparent within each and ask staff what stereotype is being expressed.

Most stereotypes regarding sexuality and aging relate to older adults not having desires, not being physically capable of having a sexual relationship, and being physically undesirable. Just as damaging is the notion that older persons who are sexually active are weird or deviant. Women who initiate relationships with younger men are labeled as "cougars" and men with younger women are seen as "dirty old men."

Research shows that even very limited education about or exposure to older adults can alleviate or eliminate common ageist beliefs.

Sexuality and Long-Term Care: Understanding and Supporting the Needs of Older Adults, by Gayle Appel Doll (Copyright 2012, by Health Professions Press, Inc.)

Barriers

Mark the described barriers to resident sexuality that you have seen in your nursing home or other senior living residence. What solution can you envision that would remove this barrier?

Barriers to Resident Sexual Expression

Barrier	Solution
Stereotypes and ageism: Staff attitudes	
Lack of privacy	
Family attitudes	
Lack of partner	
No privacy	
Other residents	

The Star Count

This activity can be used to identify which residents in the home may be experiencing isolation. Make a list of all of the residents living in the home and hang it in an area that is not accessible to them. Hand out sticky stars to each of the employees of the home, including housekeeping, maintenance, dietary, and nursing. Have the staff stick stars next to the names of the residents with whom they have meaningful interactions on a daily basis. Meaningful interaction will be defined as conversations of more than ten words and may or may not include touching depending on the desires of the resident.

This is an activity done in schools and it typically reveals a pattern in which one-third of the students have many stars, a third of the students have some stars, and a third of the students have very few stars. It stands to reason that nursing home residents would follow a similar distribution.

The third of the residents who get very few stars may not receive as much attention from staff for various reasons. They may have challenging personalities or advanced dementia. Another type of resident purposefully tries to avoid making extra work for staff; occasionally staff will be too overwhelmed with tasks to notice the quiet folks. Each staff person should select one of these persons to focus additional attention on. The care teams may choose to be specific about what "additional attention" should be (e.g., one 10-minute conversation per day).

Sexuality and Long-Term Care: Understanding and Supporting the Needs of Older Adults, by Gayle Appel Doll (Copyright 2012, by Health Professions Press, Inc.)

Staff Attitudes about Resident Sexuality

OBJECTIVES

- Describe staff attitudes toward resident sexuality
- Explore strategies for managing resident sexuality
- Discuss regulations that guide staff interventions
- Identify training strategies to change staff attitudes

Donald had transferred to Sunnydale nursing home from another home where he had been identified as a troublemaker. His reputation followed him; and staff were wary of him and avoided him when they could. Donald was visited by Lydia, the unit's social worker. In the course of her visit she asked him what might make his stay at the new facility more comfortable. He replied by saying that he would like help finding a woman to please him sexually. This shocked the social worker because she had never heard such a request. After determining that the request appeared to be legitimate rather than just made to create a reaction, Lydia decided to discuss the issue with the interdisciplinary team that was assigned to help Donald settle into the facility. The group determined that nothing illegal, such as hiring a prostitute, could be done for his specific request but that Donald appeared to have a legitimate sexual need. The team asked Lydia to learn more about his desire. When interviewed, Donald commented that he was lonely and needed a woman to make him feel satisfied. Lydia explained that this request was against the law and therefore inappropriate, but she offered alternatives to help him meet his need. The resident liked the suggestion of using sexually explicit materials for his sexual fulfillment. To address his need the team came up with a twofold solution. They purchased (with Donald's money) various materials that he could view in the privacy of his room. While reviewing his admittance documentation, the team noted that Donald had a history of sub-

The section Regulatory Considerations was contributed by Laci Cornelison, LBSW, LTCA, Research Associate, Center on Aging, Kansas State University.

stance abuse and feelings of abandonment. The team agreed to try to give extra attention to developing relationships with him. As he started feeling connected to others, he began to have fewer discussions about feeling lonely and fewer requests to view the materials.

This case story, perhaps more than any other in this book, reveals the complexity of the decisions that must be made to honor residents' sexual needs. The request goes well beyond asking a caregiver to hang a "do not disturb" sign on the door, or to knock and wait for a response before entering a room. It also goes beyond challenging old stereotypes that older people do not have sexual thoughts. In this case, the resident's request required that a staff member purchase materials that to the staff member may have seemed immoral or disturbing. Since Americans have been acculturated to believe that older adults are asexual, sexual expression within the nursing home almost always takes caregivers by surprise. Due to the scope and range of sexual expressions, each resident's needs must be handled individually. This chapter explores typical staff reactions to resident sexuality and training opportunities that can provide person-centered approaches to addressing residents' needs. This preparation can lead to more appropriate staff responses and a more sensitive environment for residents (Sidebar 3.1).

While large-scale studies regarding sexual practices of older people have become more frequently reported in the national news, most Americans are still socialized to react negatively to sex and intimacy among older adults. Images of sexuality are consistently reinforced as activities for people with young, healthy, beautiful bodies. The mere thought of parents having intercourse typically makes an adult child cringe (Sidebar 3.2). Staff may develop relationships with residents who feel like a family member, sometimes seeing the resident as a parent or a grandparent. This can create discomfort for both the resident and staff member with respect to sexual matters. Staff responses to residents may also be mediated by their own fears of aging, which makes it difficult for them to relate to older residents.

> "Nurses that hold ageist views of elderly sexuality are not providing holistic care. It is not possible to provide care that aims to maximize potential, independence, and control while denying or ridiculing a core aspect of their identity." (Nay, 1992)

STAFF ATTITUDES ABOUT OLDER ADULT SEXUALITY

Staff assumptions about the inability of residents to perform sexually are often firmly entrenched. Perhaps because of this belief new staff members are seldom

Sidebar 3.1
Sex in a Danish Nursing Home

When a male resident at a nursing home in Denmark made an indecent sexual proposal to a member of the staff, the home's director told a nurse to telephone for a prostitute.

"There was a considerable change in his demeanor after the escort girl had paid him a visit," the director said in an interview. "We do this for our clients just as we offer them other services that they need as human beings."

The leader of the Copenhagen-based Danish Sex-worker Association states on the association's website that prostitutes often visit Danish care homes for older residents. She goes on to assert that "To forbid vulnerable customers from obtaining the services of a legal business is discriminating, both against the sex workers and the people who need help to get the services."

Source: Retrieved from http://www.bloomberg.com/apps/news?pid=newsarchive&sid=aVUcop17mg7s

Sidebar 3.2
The "Ick" Response

Have you ever tried mentioning at a party or gathering a time when you caught your parents having sex? What was the response from your friends or colleagues? Did they roll their eyes, counter with "horror" stories of their own, or get the dry heaves? People have been socialized to have these reactions. Beliefs that sex among older people is disgusting are firmly entrenched and may be difficult to destroy.

trained to be aware of or to understand the sexual needs of residents. When a resident expresses him- or herself sexually, staff members are often caught by surprise and may react inappropriately (disgust, anger, horror, disbelief). These reactions may, in turn, cause a resident to feel ashamed or embarrassed or that his or her expressions of sexuality are seen as unhealthy, immoral, or unacceptable by staff.

Wendy, a new certified nursing assistant (CNA) at Sunnyriver Home, knocked on Clarence's door but, as she had observed in other nursing staff, did not wait for a response before entering. Walking into the room she was surprised to find that Clarence was not alone in bed. Not waiting to find out who his guest might be, Wendy shrieked and rushed out the door to find Donna, the charge nurse. The door was left wide open, and Clarence and his guest were left feeling humiliated and unhappy. What might have been a better response?

Kansas State University Center on Aging conducted a survey of Kansas nursing home administrators and social service workers of how they felt staff would react to sexual expression among residents. Figure 3.1 shows some of the results. Survey participants could choose more than one response. The majority (69%) said that staff would ask a supervisor if they were aware of any sexual activity. Other popular responses were to follow the facility policy (41%) and try to respectfully help the resident (51%), both of which are surprising given that later questions revealed that few homes had policies or training that might help staff members respond appropriately and effectively. Fewer (32%) said they would respond with disgust, ignore the issue (28%), or panic (20%). Nearly all of the short-answer responses to this question indicated that a staff member would check with someone else or would "redirect the resident." These responses reveal that staff more often view sexual expression among residents as nonnormative and as a problem that must be treated.

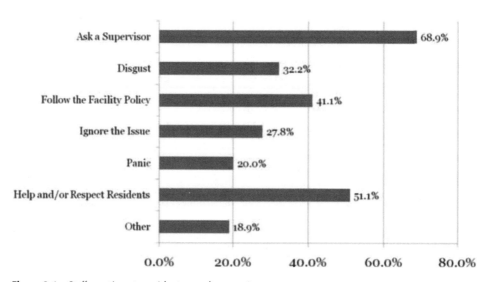

Figure 3.1   Staff reactions to resident sexual expression

The answers also indicate a lack of training, as evidenced by staff members choosing to consult with a supervisor rather than addressing a situation on their own.

TYPES OF SEXUAL EXPRESSION IN LONG-TERM CARE AS IDENTIFIED BY STAFF

Caregivers generally identify three types of sexual expression in nursing homes—love and caring, romance, and eroticism. *Love and caring* indicate strong affection or attraction between two residents. *Romance* signifies a scope of emotions that idealizes objects of affection. Feelings of sexual excitement or desire denote *eroticism* and may result in intercourse. Ehrenfeld and colleagues (1997) interviewed caregivers and found that each of the three types of sexual expression elicited profoundly different reactions. Caregivers were sympathetic toward love and caring. These types of relationships may be between really good friends and even potentially between two people of the same sex. These residents take care of each other or simply provide a level of intimacy that is otherwise missing from their lives. Staff might find these relationships "cute" and may find ways to foster and support them.

> Sarah and Eloise have been roommates for 2 and a half years and they are inseparable. They hold hands as they wait for meals and can be seen stroking each other's hair, especially during times of stress.

Romance might be the source of amusement among staff. The romantic relationship might be likened to how one might feel about a son's first junior high school girlfriend—it is cute, as long as it does not lead to a sexual relationship. Staff may feel comfortable encouraging and supporting a romantic relationship among residents, as long as it remains nonsexual.

> Dorothy and Bob lived in the dementia care unit at Sunnydale Home. Neither could remember the other's name, but they knew that they cared for each other and could be found holding hands in the dayroom all day long, sometimes without ever saying a word. The staff knew that if ever one of the two was unhappy or restless, they could find the other and all would be well with the world.

Of the three types of sexual expression, eroticism evokes a range of emotional responses on the part of staff, including confusion, embarrassment, helplessness, anger, denial, and aversion. Sexual desire or excitement reaches beyond the comfort zone of most caregivers.

> Mavis, a CNA at Sunnybrook Hills, complained to her friend, "I had to remove Charlie from the living room again because he was playing with himself. The way I feel about it is this: I know my son does it, but as long as he does it when I don't have to know about it, it's OK."

Staff, who may harbor paternalistic feelings toward some residents, may overreact to sexual situations by treating those in their care as children.

Sexual Expression and Gender Differences

Staff appear to differentiate sexual activity by gender, believing that men are more likely to express themselves sexually than are women (Archibald, 1998). They tend to view sexual expressions negatively and are more likely to report them to medical professionals, thinking the behaviors are inappropriate or pathological. Transferring a male resident to another wing is a common intervention. In other words, male residents are seen as "dirty old men" when they attempt to express themselves sexually. On the other hand, staff either tend to overlook female sexual expression or feel compelled to protect a female resident (Nay, 1992). A female resident's sexuality is seldom seen as an active threat to other residents, and is more of a concern in light of the masculine attention she may attract (Activity 3.1). According to Ward, Vass, Aggarwal, Garfield, and Cybyk (2005, p. 5), "Masculine sexual transgression contrasts with feminine vulnerability, often generating a punish/protect response within care settings."

STAFF RESPONSES TO SEXUAL EXPRESSION

To be successful, a long-term care organization must promote efficiency. Established routines regulate all resident activities from mealtimes to toileting, bathing, recreational activities, and sleeping. Scheduled routines limit the range of options available to residents. Residents begin to understand that their adherence to these schedules is necessary for the smooth operation of the facility, and they become reluctant to ask for anything that might disrupt the flow of routine. In their own efforts not to disrupt established routines or interrupt their ability to provide efficient care, staff may not give much importance to assisting residents in fulfilling their sexual needs. Residents' reluctance to voice requests or complaints can also influence the amount of respect caregivers give to the right to privacy. If residents do not express or assert a right to privacy, caregivers assume that residents are not concerned about breaches of privacy. And while caregivers may perceive that privacy is important, they believe the lack of it is less important than the physical health of the residents.

Most of the literature on sexuality in nursing homes indicates that staff have a limited understanding of how to manage sexual activity among older adults. Frequently the behavior is seen as deviant, abnormal, and problematic rather than as an expression of love and intimacy. Staff may respond by punishing a resident or with apathy or hostility toward residents who express or act on a need for sexual intimacy or lament the loss of such intimacy. Others may simply ignore the behavior, perhaps hoping that it will go away.

Roach (2004) distinguished four common staff responses to resident sexuality, each of which affects residents differently:

1. *Standing guard* occurs when staff address situations in ways to prevent themselves from feeling uncomfortable. Staff who adopt this approach do so to avoid having to deal with residents' sexuality and do not acknowledge or address their sexual needs. This approach may result in a lower quality of life and health declines in residents, and is typical in homes where residents' sexuality is strongly discouraged (Roach, 2004).

   At Goldenroad Manor caregivers keep a watchful eye on residents. If new relationships develop, residents are separated before they can become too intimate.

2. *Reactive protection* also avoids staff uneasiness with resident sexuality. Staff abide by their individual moral, religious, or cultural values to "protect" residents. This approach is potentially more harmful to residents than standing guard due to the differences in values among staff as well as any potential staff hidden agendas. In a nursing home culture where residents' sexuality is supported, staff are less likely to be able to create reactive barriers for residents. A paternalistic approach, mentioned earlier, falls under the category of reactive protection as another means of controlling sexual expression. Sometimes staff think of and treat residents as if they were children, encouraging them to refrain from sexual activity.

The person-centered policy at Sunset Towers supports resident sexuality. However, many of the staff members feel that out-of-wedlock relationships are morally wrong and potentially harmful to the residents. They do what they can to prevent intimacy and sexual activities between residents.

3. *Guarding the guards* occurs when staff come up with and implement an approach to addressing a resident's sexuality and sexual needs that is not accepted by other staff within a restrictive nursing home environment. Staff have discussed resident rights and responsibilities, including the right to sexual expression, and guard residents' rights to intimacy from other staff members.

   At Sunrise Manor staff are told to strictly prevent residents from becoming intimately involved. But when John and Clara started spending time together, several of their caregivers found ways to encourage the relationship. The secrecy added excitement to the ordinary life of the nursing home, and the staff felt like they were living their own reality television drama.

4. Management can choose to take a proactive protection approach by training and educating staff about resident sexuality as well as strategies to respond to residents' needs in a dignified, respectful, and consistent manner. This approach produces positive outcomes for both residents and staff. Staff do not suppress resident sexuality and feel more comfortable dealing with diverse forms of sexual expression due to their increased awareness and sensitivity to the needs of residents.

   Newly hired CNA Wendy walked in on Clarence and his guest. She quickly assessed the situation and removed herself, closing the door quietly behind her. She made a note to herself to report the incident to the social worker so that Clarence and his friend could be provided with education about protection.

Of the four common staff responses to resident sexuality, *proactive protection* creates the best outcomes for all involved; however, it requires careful thought and planning. Staff need to be trained to have an appropriate response; there should be no assumption that residents will react appropriately without some type of intervention (Activity 3.2).

When Staff Inadvertently Encourage Resident Sexual Behavior

Caregiver staff may also inadvertently encourage sexual behaviors on the part of residents. For example, caregivers may choose not to report some inappropriate behaviors so that they can avoid being blamed or even laughed at by their peers. Or a caregiver, thinking he or she is simply being attentive to a resident, may banter in a teasing manner, such as "Oh, Carl, you're such a ladies' man!" The resident might construe such a comment as an invitation for or tacit approval of a sexual advance either toward another resident or toward a staff member. Staff who dress provocatively may receive unwanted advances. Some nursing homes, in an attempt to provide quality-of-life experiences for residents, might hold a "bar night," which may lead to disinhibited behaviors and possible sexual advances toward staff members or other residents.

Resident sexual advances toward staff may lead to turnover. Most of the CNAs who provide intimate care for residents are young women. If these individuals are not trained to recognize types of sexual expression, understand the underlying causes of residents' behaviors, and address inappropriate behaviors, they may feel more inclined to leave the home rather than endure any awkwardness or frustrations.

Management Responses to Sexual Expression

Administrators and managers have a lot of knowledge about older adult sexuality, as measured by survey responses. They also tend to have more restrictive attitudes about resident sexuality than direct caregivers. Low, Lui, Lee, Thompson, and Chau (2005) found that nursing home leaders will allow sexual behavior when it is privately expressed, considered culturally safe, and not difficult to manage. Hand holding might be seen as acceptable while other sexual expressions are seen as less acceptable when displayed in public or when a caregiver is present. What management deem appropriate expressions of physical intimacy may be limited to hand holding or hugs or to social activities such as dancing. Restrictive measures imposed by administrators and managers may arise from a need to see that the organization runs smoothly, avoiding problems among other residents and families of residents.

STAFF TOLERANCE OF RESIDENT SEXUALITY

It is rather interesting to note that a study done in 1999 (Bauer) found that staff members were far more tolerant of sexual behaviors in the nursing home than were the residents themselves and their family members. These behaviors included masturbation, engaging in sexual activity, viewing sexual materials, and making a sexual advance toward a staff member. Despite the fact that staff members find some behaviors more acceptable than others, the sexuality of residents is still seen as a concern and a burden. Due to limited insights and understanding of older adult sexuality, nursing home staff often view sexual activity as behavior problems rather than expressions of love and intimacy. Staff cope with their feelings about resident sexuality through humor, ridicule, and teasing. Caregivers may use humor to communicate more easily about sexuality, which allows them to relieve the stress of the situation. If used with sensitivity, humor can be an effective strategy for safely dealing with activities and behaviors that staff may find too emotionally and socially unacceptable to address directly. Conversely, humor may have the effect of coercing residents to conform to ageist beliefs that older adults are asexual and should, therefore, conceal their genuine needs (Activity 3.3). An example might be to tell a resident, "Aren't you too old to have a girlfriend?"

FEDERAL REGULATORY CONSIDERATIONS

Nursing home staff and administration must comply with federal regulations and guidelines that direct the way they deliver care, specifically those issued by the Centers for Medicare and Medicaid Services (CMS). This section highlights federal guidelines that support (and sometimes inhibit) sexual expression. Each home must also be aware of state mandates that may add further instruction.

Currently, there are no federal regulations that specifically address sexual activity and residents in the nursing home. CMS, however, has issued several F-Tag regulations (short for "Federal Tags") that provide guidance for long-term care facilities when situations arise. For example, F-Tag 175 (483.10 (m)), Married Couples, states that, "The resident has the right to share a room with his or her spouse when married residents live in the same facility and both spouses consent to the arrangement." The CMS interpretive guidelines acknowledge that this regulation does not give married couples or facilities the right to ask another resident to relocate to accommodate the couple. When a room becomes available, the facility must permit the couple to share the room if they choose. Furthermore, this regulation does not prohibit the facility from accommodating residents who wish to room with another nursing home resident of their choice.

The issue of privacy also directly impacts sexual activity. F-Tag 164 (483.10 (e)), Privacy and Confidentiality of Personal and Clinical Records, defines a right to personal privacy, including with respect to accommodations, medical treatment, written communications, personal care, visits, and meetings of family and resident groups. Residents have the right to privacy and to have their needs met, as long as those rights do not infringe on other residents' needs and rights.

> "Right to personal privacy" means that the resident has the right to privacy with whomever the resident wishes to be private and that this privacy should include full visual, and, to the extent desired, for visits or other activities, auditory privacy. Private space may be created flexibly and need not be dedicated solely for visitation purposes. (F-Tag 164 (483.10(e)), CMS Interpretive Guidelines)

F-Tag 241 (483.15 (a)), Dignity, states that a facility must "promote care for residents in a manner and in an environment that maintains or enhances each resident's dignity and respect in full recognition of his or her individuality." This includes respecting residents' private space and property by knocking on doors and requesting permission to enter, as well as closing doors at the resident's request.

F-Tag 454 (483.70 (d)), Physical Environment, defines privacy within the resident's room. It states that resident rooms must be "designed and equipped for adequate nursing care, comfort, and privacy of residents." F-Tag 460, Full Visual Privacy, requires room designs (e.g., ceiling-suspended curtains) that ensure the full visual privacy of residents. According to the CMS Interpretive Guidelines, *full visual privacy* means that

> residents have a means of completely withdrawing from public view while occupying their bed (e.g., curtain, moveable screens, private room). The guidelines do not intend to limit the provisions of privacy to solely one or more curtains, movable screens or a private room. Facility operators are free to use other means to provide full visual privacy, with those means varying according to the needs and requests of residents. (F-Tag 460 (483.70(d)(1)(iv), CMS Interpretive Guidelines)

Although the regulation does not spell out specific means for providing full visual privacy, the requirement explicitly states that measures must be in place to address the need for privacy within a resident's room.

The degree to which staff members respect the privacy of residents varies from home to home. Residents are dependent on the attitudes and actions of staff for the provision of privacy, but not all caregivers comply with the appropriate protocol. Also, staff often do not view protecting the privacy of residents regarding intimacy and sexuality as part of the caregiving role. Furthermore, the provision of privacy may not fit comfortably into the model of efficiency that most caregiving institutions adopt. As mentioned earlier, mealtimes, bathing, sleeping, and recreational activities are regimented routines that staff are reluctant to disrupt in their efforts to provide efficient care. Residents are expected to adhere to these routines with the appropriate behavior.

Resident autonomy and choice also play a role in addressing sexual activity in the nursing home. F-Tag 242 (483.15 (b)), Self-Determination and Participation, states that the resident has a right to "make choices about aspects of his or her life in the facility that are significant to the resident." This regulation supports resident autonomy related to choices in activities, schedules, or forms of bathing. It is the facility's responsibility to create an environment that respects residents' right to exercise their autonomy and to provide the necessary assistance to help residents fulfill their choices. This regulation suggests that a resident has the right to choose to room with a person of the resident's choice if both consent.

Closely related to issues of self-determination, F-Tag 246, Accommodation of Needs, states that a resident has the right to "reside and receive service in the facility with reasonable accommodation of individual needs and preferences, except when the health or safety of the individual or other residents would be endangered." According to the Interpretive Guidelines, "this includes making adaptations of the resident's bedroom and bathroom furniture and fixtures." The guidelines further state that bedroom furniture should be arranged in accordance with the resident's preferences whenever possible. When applied to accommodating residents' need for intimacy and sexual expression, this regulation may impact a resident's ability to share a bed with a partner or to arrange a room so that beds are next to each other.

F-Tag 279, Comprehensive Care Plans, unites the rights of self-determination and accommodation of needs. It states, "The facility must develop a comprehensive care plan for each resident that includes measurable objectives and timetables to meet a resident's medical, nursing, and mental and psychosocial needs that are identified in the comprehensive assessment." Sexual activity may be identified as a need to be included in the comprehensive care plan. This regulation pushes facilities to provide services that "maintain the resident's highest level of practicable physical, mental, and psychosocial well-being." Accommodating the sexual needs of a resident can assist in maintaining his or her highest level of well-being. Residents should be involved in the care planning process as much as their level of functioning permits, including those with cognitive impairments that affect their decision-making capacity.

Of final consideration is the issue of sexual abuse. F-Tag 223, Abuse, states that all residents are to be free from verbal, sexual, physical, and mental abuse. The regulation defines sexual abuse as "sexual harassment, sexual coercion, or sexual assault." In order to comply with this regulation, facilities have a responsibility to develop and implement written policies and procedures that prohibit abuse and for screening and training employees to protect residents from abuse, as called for by F-Tag 224 (Mistreatment, Neglect, or Misappropriation of Resident Property) and F-Tag 226 (Staff Treatment of Residents: Policies and Procedures). The purpose is to assure that the facility is doing all that is within its control to prevent incidents of sexual abuse. Facility procedures must include policies that address

- Screening
- Training prevention
- Identification
- Investigation
- Protection
- Reporting/response

Due to the complexity of some issues, it may be necessary to consult a state surveyor, who may be able to help answer specific questions or refer questions to the state ombudsman program. Ombudsmen serve as advocates on issues affecting older residents living in nursing homes. As mentioned in Chapter 1, the Omnibus Reconciliation Act of 1987 and other amendments define the ombudsmen as advocates who help prevent abuse, neglect, and exploitation of older individuals. Long-term care ombudsmen are resident advocates who serve as negotiators, problem solvers, educators, objective investigators, and collaborators. In situations where a solution is not clear, ombudsmen can help facilities and residents achieve an equitable resolution (Activity 3.4).

CHANGING STAFF ATTITUDES THROUGH TRAINING

Fortunately, staff attitudes appear to be relatively easy to change. Training programs that focus on debunking myths about older adult sexuality have been successful in helping caregivers to recognize sexuality as a basic human need that does not disappear with age (Jankowiak, 2008; Kennedy, Haque, & Zarankow, 1997).

One tool to incorporate into a training program is Maslow's hierarchy of five basic human needs (Maslow, 1970). Portrayed graphically as a pyramid (see Figure 3.2), sex falls within the lower level of basic human needs (physiological) and appears again as sexual intimacy at the third level (love and belonging). The pyramid can be used to increase staff understanding of human needs. If a nursing home is providing person-centered care, there is an inherent understanding of this theory and of the concept of sexuality as a basic need of all humans.

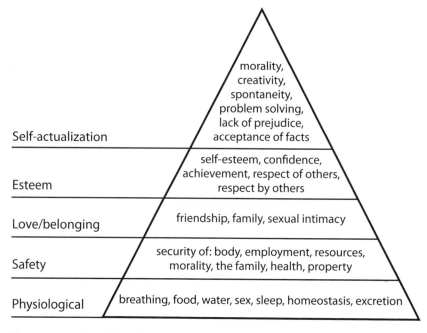

Figure 3.2   Maslow's hierarchy of human needs.

Another tool that can be helpful in discussions related to sexuality in nursing homes is the Staff Attitudes about Intimacy and Dementia (SAID) survey (Kuhn, 2002). This instrument can be used to measure staff beliefs and attitudes as well as provide a good starting point for education and training (Sidebar 3.3).

Caregivers may perceive resident sexual expression as problematic or inappropriate behavior when viewed through their own moral lens. One very specific way to begin to change these attitudes is for staff to avoid placing notes about resident masturbation or use of pornography in care charts or to avoid raising these issues at team meetings unless the information is absolutely essential to the care of the resident. Staff should honor residents' privacy in these matters.

With respect to residents with dementia, staff should be taught that the behavioral effects of frontal lobe degeneration—loss of social judgment, diminished impulse control, and a lack of understanding of the consequences of sexual acts—are not willful acting out, mischief, or malice. Many of these behaviors are seen as problematic when they occur in public spaces. Unfortunately, there are few private places in nursing homes, so caregivers need to be taught strategies to divert residents to other activities. Staff should also be trained that inappropriate or ill-timed expressions of sexuality may represent an unfulfilled need for intimacy that can come from close personal relationships. Staff should be encouraged to develop caring relationships with residents that may help fulfill the need for intimacy. (See

Sidebar 3.3
Staff Attitudes about Intimacy and Dementia (SAID) Survey

The following statements are intended to reveal your attitudes about intimacy and sexuality issues that arise among persons with dementia living in residential care facilities. Circle the numbered response that best suits your viewpoint. 1 = Strongly agree, 2 = Somewhat agree, 3 = Somewhat disagree, 4 = Strongly disagree. You do not have to share your responses with anyone.

Competent and consenting residents who are married are entitled to be sexually intimate with their spouse in a private place within a care facility.

1   2   3   4

Competent and consenting residents who are single are entitled to be sexually intimate with each other in a care facility.

1   2   3   4

Competent and consenting residents who are married, but not to each other, are entitled to be sexually intimate with one another in a care facility.

1   2   3   4

A married couple with one spouse living in the community and the other one with dementia residing in a care facility is entitled to be sexually intimate in a private place within the facility.

1   2   3   4

Residents who have dementia are not capable of making sound decisions regarding participation in sexual relationships.

1   2   3   4

(continued on next page)

Sidebar 3.3 (continued)

A married couple, with one spouse living at home and one with dementia residing in a care facility, is entitled to be sexually intimate even though the one with dementia appears to be unable to give consent.

1   2   3   4

A spouse living in the community is entitled to become intimately involved with someone else if his or her spouse has dementia and resides in a care facility.

1   2   3   4

Two residents, both of whom have dementia, are entitled to an exclusive and consensual relationship but should not be sexually intimate if one of them is married to another person.

1   2   3   4

Two residents, one with Alzheimer's disease and the other who is cognitively intact, are entitled to be sexually intimate as long as they are both single and their relationship appears consensual.

1   2   3   4

Two residents, both of whom are single and have dementia, are entitled to be sexually intimate if their relationship appears consensual and their family members do not object.

1   2   3   4

Two residents, both of whom are single and have dementia, are entitled to be sexually intimate if their relationship appears consensual, although one confuses the other for a deceased spouse.

1   2   3   4

A resident with dementia is entitled to be sexually intimate with two different residents as long as there is no sign of coercion in these relationships.

1   2   3   4

Sidebar 3.3 (continued)

A resident is entitled to masturbate in private as long as his or her personal safety is ensured.

1   2   3   4

Two residents who are of the same sex are entitled to a close friendship, but sexual activity between them is unacceptable.

1   2   3   4

Staff should provide a private place so as to allow a male and female resident to engage in sexual activity as long as both of them are cognitively intact.

1   2   3   4

Staff should provide a private place so as to allow a male and a female resident to engage in sexual activity, even though both of them are mildly impaired due to dementia.

1   2   3   4

If family members object to a relative with dementia having sexual relations with others, it is the duty of the staff to prevent such activity.

1   2   3   4

A resident displaying hypersexual behavior should be transferred out of the facility.

1   2   3   4

No one should interfere in the sexual lives of residents as long as no civil or criminal laws are broken.

1   2   3   4

Source: Kuhn, D. (2002). Intimacy, sexuality, and residents with dementia. *Alzheimer's Care Quarterly, 3*(2), 165–176. Reprinted with permission.

Chapters 5, Dementia, and 6, Inappropriate Behaviors, for additional strategies for diverting residents from inappropriate behaviors.)

Staff training should also address the importance of touch, that humans have a need for personal touch—to be held, hugged, patted, and caressed. Many nursing home residents are surrounded by people, yet they can feel lonely and in need of intimacy, including through touch. Caregivers should, however, never assume that every resident wants to be touched. As discussed in Chapter 2, when staff are consistently assigned to the same small group of residents they become better acquainted with their needs and can learn how to appropriately touch a resident.

ELEMENTS OF A STAFF TRAINING PROGRAM

Single-offering trainings have been shown to promote changes in staff attitudes. In a training developed by the Kansas State University Center on Aging, caregivers are sensitized to understand sexuality as a basic human need (Jankowiak, 2008). To challenge and change their assumptions, staff learn facts about sexuality in aging populations, examine the types of sexual expression, and explore strategies for redirecting inappropriate sexual activity. Staff also examine case studies and are given the opportunity to tell their own stories of successful strategies to promote resident sexuality. Six weeks after training staff members reported in focus groups that they were much more likely to view resident intimacy and sexuality as positives and had taken steps to provide privacy for residents (hanging a do-not-disturb sign on a resident's door, waiting for a response before entering a room after knocking, finding activities outside the room for a roommate while a couple shares private time).

Training materials should be relevant and appropriate to the types of sexual expression staff encounter on a regular basis. Staff training should promote empathy. Simulations and experiential activities that require the caregiver to live as a resident enhance understanding of how residents live in an institutional environment.

One training strategy is to develop a systematic approach to presenting sexual incidents, which may include decision trees or worksheets that systematically document sexual behavior, caregivers' personal beliefs about the issue, and choices of actions suggested by peers and supervisors.

A model proposed for developing nurses' skills for working with sexual expression in residents goes by the name RESPECT (Lorenz, 2009):

Resources. Nurses should learn as much as they can about older adult sexuality, and they should provide resources (i.e., reading materials) for older adults. Left in waiting rooms, these materials will leave the impression that it is okay to discuss this subject.

Education. Give residents information about the physical changes with aging that affect sexuality. Include education about sexually transmitted diseases, including HIV.

Support. Support the right of residents to express themselves sexually and act as a resident advocate with other health care professionals.

Protection. Protect residents who are unable to make their own decisions about engaging in sexual activity. Also, protect residents from their own inappropriate behavior by implementing strategies to distract, divert, or attend to the need that the resident may be expressing (see Chapter 6).

Empowerment. Encourage healthy forms of sexual expression among residents. Help them to feel attractive with trips to the beauty salon or by assisting them with their grooming and clothing.

Confidentiality. Respect the privacy of residents and remove barriers to sexual expression. Find ways to accommodate conjugal visits or encourage home visits. Wait for a response after knocking before entering a resident's room and close the door after entering or leaving.

Tactfulness. At admission, ask a new resident about his or her preferred types of sexual expression in a respectful and tactful manner. Leave the door open for continued discussion, and do not come off as hurrying or prying. This subject may be difficult for some older adults, especially if their children are present. Get permission before sharing any resident information given in private.

Perhaps the most important goal of training is that it should occur before a staff member actually witnesses a resident sexually expressing him- or herself. Few new CNAs have received training in this area in their certification courses. Facilities should provide information during the new staff member's orientation about resident sexual needs and how caregivers are expected to respond to resident sexuality.

Providing training opportunities for staff at the nursing home acknowledges the administration's support. A training initiative can evolve into a regularly scheduled in-service through which staff can generate their own agendas for regular discussions of sexual issues specific to their home. Staff may take ownership of the training and help to individualize strategies for their resident population. (See Activities 3.5 and 3.6 for personal and group activities that explore staff attitudes toward resident sexuality.)

DISCUSSION

Returning to the story at the beginning of the chapter, Lydia, the social worker, was initially shocked by Donald's request. Had she received some training from the facility about the possibility that a request like this might occur and had she been given information about organization policies related to such a request, she might not have had such a strong reaction.

Lydia had, however, been trained to expect the unexpected. She did not lose control of the situation or overreact. She examined the request and determined that accommodating it would be illegal. She also recognized that the request represented a human need for sexual expression and intimacy. Setting aside her own embarrassment, Lydia took the appropriate steps to work with Donald to identify a legal and acceptable solution to address his needs (using his money to purchase pornographic materials for him). In addition, she did not work in isolation, instead consulting with an interdisciplinary team to determine the best options for Donald. Nursing home policies should identify who should be on the team and their respective roles. Policies that allow staff to purchase sexual aids or materials for residents need to be sensitive to the feelings of staff members and should not force them to do something that makes them feel uncomfortable.

As part of her "detective" work, Lydia learned from the interdisciplinary team that Donald came to the facility with a history of substance abuse and feelings of abandonment. This may have triggered further assessments for clinical depression, adjustment disorders, and any other category of psychiatric illness that may require appropriate professional intervention. The team, which had been trained in the person-centered care model, ventured to try a behavioral approach of giving Donald extra attention to develop relationships with him, which seemed to have a successful outcome (Donald expressed that he felt less lonely and made fewer requests for pornographic materials).

Perhaps the most significant outcome from these interventions was that Donald's needs were honored. He was not ignored or punished, and in honoring his desires the staff grew to understand Donald better and became his friends.

In a study that measured the effects of sexuality training on nursing home caregivers, staff expressed mixed feelings about their roles (Walker & Harrington, 2002). While they believed that residents had the right to do whatever they wanted in the privacy of their own rooms, they did not feel obligated to help residents obtain items such as erotic videos, pornography, or condoms. Only 21% of those surveyed said they would purchase condoms for sexually active residents, even though they were aware that this population is at high risk for sexually transmitted diseases.

Can you think of other ways that Lydia and her team could have managed the situation? How do you think the staff or administration at your facility would have addressed this situation? What other scenarios of resident sexual expression can you think of, and how might they be managed by staff in your long-term care setting?

SUMMARY

Long-term care staff must walk a thin line that separates protecting residents and helping them to attain their highest level of functioning. This charge may become difficult to honor for those residents who wish to be able to express themselves sexually. Not only must caregivers address residents' needs, they must also balance this intention with helping to meet the organization's needs. These needs may include protecting the organization against prosecution, honoring other residents' care needs and dignity, and getting their work done efficiently and effectively.

This chapter provides staff with information to make informed decisions in managing resident sexuality. Caregivers must first challenge their own biases and beliefs about older adult sexuality. Staff training programs can debunk myths about older adult sexuality, teach caregivers to recognize sexuality as a basic human need that does not disappear with age, promote strategies to assist staff in honoring the needs of residents.

REFERENCES

Archibald, C. (1998). Sexuality, dementia and residential care: Managers report and response. *Health and Social Care in the Community, 6*(2), 95–101.

Bauer, M. (1999). Their only privacy is between their sheets: Privacy and the sexuality of elderly nursing home residents. *Journal of Gerontological Nursing, 25*(8), 37–41.

Ehrenfeld, M., Tabak, N., Bronner, G., & Bergman, R. (1997). Ethical dilemmas concerning sexuality of elderly patients suffering from dementia. *International Journal of Nursing Practice, 3*(4), 255–259.

Jankowiak, M. (2008). Sexuality in nursing facilities: Awareness of residents' needs for intimacy improves caregivers' understanding of the issue and dispels some myths about old age. *Provider, 35*(1), 33–35.

Kennedy, G.J., Haque, M., & Zarankow, B. (1997). Human sexuality in late life. *International Journal of Mental Health, 26,* 35–46.

Kuhn, D. (2002). Intimacy, sexuality, and residents with dementia. *Alzheimer's Care Quarterly, 3*(2), 165–176.

Lorenz, J. (2009) When is old too old? *Advance for Long-Term Care Management.* Retrieved from http://long-term-care.advanceweb.com/Articlesex-and-the-older-adult.aspx.

Low, L., Lui, M., Lee, D., Thompson, D., & Chau, J. (2005). Promoting awareness of sexuality of older people in residential care. *Electronic Journal of Human Sexuality, 8,* 1–12. Retrieved from http://www.ejhs.org/volume8/sexuality_of_older_people.html.

Maslow, A. (1970). *Motivation and personality.* New York: Harper & Row.

Nay, R. (1992). Sexuality and aged women in nursing homes. *Geriatric Nursing, 13*(6), 312–314.

Roach, S. M. (2004). Sexual behavior of nursing home residents: Staff perceptions and responses. *Journal of Advanced Nursing, 48*(4), 371–378.

Walker, B. L., & Harrington, D. (2002). Effects of staff training on staff knowledge and attitudes about sexuality. *Educational Gerontology, 28*(8), 639–654.

Ward, R., Vass, A., Aggarwal, N., Garfield, C., & Cybyk, B. (2005). A kiss is still a kiss? The construction of sexuality in dementia care. *Dementia. 4*(1), 49–73.

Discussion Questions

Think about the last time you witnessed a resident sexual expression. Was it initiated by a male or a female? How did you feel about the expression? Would you have felt differently if it had been a sexual expression made by a resident of another gender? Do you think males get a "bad rap," or is the "dirty old man" reputation sometimes deserved?

For insight into the reasons for the behavior see Chapter 6.

Where Do We Fit?

Begin a discussion on policies related to sexuality by assessing the approaches of the organization and its members. In small groups hand out the definition of each of the four common staff responses to resident sexuality listed in the text. Have the group vote on which approach best fits their own organization. Count the votes for all of the groups, and lead a discussion about the results. What changes will be needed to institute a proactive protection approach?

Discussion

Think of examples where humor has been used to cope with resident sexual expression. Can you think of times when humor was harmful? When humor was used effectively?

Care Planning for Sexual Expression

How would you write a plan of care that addresses sexual expression? Here's one story and a corresponding sample care plan (see next page):

At Oak Grove Life Care Center, staff members have noticed that two residents seem to be forming a romantic relationship with one another. Mary Ellen is an 85-year-old woman who has been a widow for 15 years. She moved into the care facility 2 years ago after having broken her hip. Joe, 82 years old, moved in 3 months ago after a recurrence of a chronic lung condition. Joe lost his wife to cancer a year ago. Both Mary Ellen and Joe are considered legally competent to make decisions for themselves.

Mary Ellen and Joe met at a facility Christmas party shortly after Joe moved in. They instantly had a connection and began spending time together each day. Staff began to notice that they were holding hands, sharing secrets, and giving each other the occasional "see you later" kiss.

One afternoon, Joe's daughter came to visit. She found Joe in his room, in bed with Mary Ellen. Joe's daughter was shocked. She slammed the door and headed straight to the administrator's office, where she complained that her father and Mary Ellen were being foolish and should not behave in such a way. She told the administrator, "Dad is too old to be starting a romance. How could he betray Mom like that?"

Sexuality and Long-Term Care: Understanding and Supporting the Needs of Older Adults, by Gayle Appel Doll (Copyright 2012, by Health Professions Press, Inc.)

Care Plan

Problem/Strength	Intervention	Evaluation
Strength: Mary Ellen finds support and comfort through a romantic relationship with another resident, Joe.	• Honor Mary Ellen's privacy as requested. • Knock before entering Mary Ellen's room. • Mary Ellen requires assistance putting down the shades in her room. Provide assistance with this as needed. • Ensure that all staff members have received sensitivity training related to older adults' sexuality. • Nursing will discuss with Mary Ellen options to protect herself from sexually transmitted diseases and assist her in obtaining protection of her choice if she desires it. • Nursing will discuss Mary Ellen's sexual health and provide treatment as needed. • All staff will offer support as needs or concerns arise within Mary Ellen's relationship with Joe. • Staff will assist Mary Ellen with scheduling and getting to beauty shop appointments.	Mary Ellen will express satisfaction with the level of staff support available to maintain her desired level of interaction with Joe over the next review period.
Problem: Mary Ellen is concerned about Joe's family's discomfort with their romantic relationship.	• Staff members will provide support and advocacy for Mary Ellen as requested. • Social work staff will provide Joe's family with educational resources as appropriate. • Social work staff will offer mediation between Mary Ellen and Joe and Joe's family if desired by either resident. • Staff will encourage Mary Ellen to engage in meaningful activity and continue pursuits to build relationships with other residents. • Staff will provide emotional support for Mary Ellen to talk about the situation if desired. • Social work staff will provide Mary Ellen contact information for the state Ombudsmen Program.	Mary Ellen will continue her relationship with Joe if she desires over the next review period.

Sexuality and Long-Term Care: Understanding and Supporting the Needs of Older Adults, by Gayle Appel Doll (Copyright 2012, by Health Professions Press, Inc.)

Your Turn

Being able to support resident sexuality requires that you examine your own beliefs and values. Consider the following situations and how each would make you feel.

- Two residents holding hands
- Two same-sex residents holding hands
- A male resident touching your breast when you bathe him
- A female resident wanting to look nice for a male resident
- Walking in on a resident masturbating in his or her room
- Observing a resident masturbating in the front living room
- A resident with dementia falling in love with another resident while her husband is still living
- A resident who views pornography repeatedly
- Two unmarried residents having intercourse

Answer the following questions:

1. How do your personal values, formed while you were growing up, affect your feelings about these situations?

_____

_____

_____

_____

2. How would you define your role as a caregiver? Do you think of yourself as a protector, a helper, an assistant, or a guide? How does the way you view your role influence your feelings about resident sexuality?

_____

_____

_____

_____

3. What would you do if you were confronted with any of these situations?

_____

_____

_____

_____

A Tupperware Party

Divide a group of at least twenty staff into two smaller groups.
The groups should be separated to different parts of the room or two
different rooms. Each small group will receive different instructions on
preprinted slips of paper. They are not to know that their instructions are
different. Two facilitators will guide discussion related to the instructions.
After about 10 minutes the groups will be brought together for a group
discussion. At this point they will be unaware that they were working
off separate instructions. The questions for the large group discussion
can be written on a board or shown on a slide.

INSTRUCTIONS FOR GROUP ONE

A resident has asked you if you would help her organize a Tupperware
party in the home. She wants to invite some of her community-living
friends as well as some of the residents in the nursing home. Would
you be willing to help? What steps would you take to prepare for
this activity? Can you think of any reasons why this activity should be
prevented?

INSTRUCTIONS FOR GROUP TWO

A resident has asked you if you would help her organize a sex toy
party in the home. She wants to invite some of her community-living

friends as well as some of the residents in the nursing home. Would you be willing to help? What steps would you take to prepare for this activity? Can you think of any reasons why this activity should be prevented?

QUESTIONS TO POST FOR LARGE GROUP DISCUSSION

- How do you feel about the resident hosting this party?
- What role would you play in facilitating the party?
- How do you think this party will be received by other residents in the facility or household?
- As a staff member, do you see any potential concerns related to this party? What are they?
- How would you try to resolve these concerns?

It may take a little while, but then it may eventually occur to staff that they are working off different instructions. This activity encourages staff to think about and discuss more openly how sexuality can fit into a person-centered culture.

Sexuality and Long-Term Care: Understanding and Supporting the Needs of Older Adults, by Gayle Appel Doll (Copyright 2012, by Health Professions Press, Inc.)

Family Influences on Resident Sexuality

OBJECTIVES

- Discuss the feelings that families experience when they move their loved one into a long-term care home

- Outline strategies for shared rooms for spouses

- Explore the role of family influence on resident sexuality

- Review legal ramifications of family influences on resident sexuality

- Discuss strategies for working with family members

Ben walked into his 95-year-old father Bob's assisted living room to find him in bed with his 82-year-old girlfriend, Dorothy. Both were residents, and they had been diagnosed as being in the early stages of dementia. Ben was irate and insisted that the staff keep the couple apart.

The incident threw the nursing home into turmoil. Ben believed that Dorothy had been the aggressor and told the staff that he thought sexual activity would be bad for his father's heart. The private nurse assigned to Bob had been supportive of the relationship when it was in the "cute" stage of handholding, but when it became sexual she "lost her senses" for religious reasons. She asked the staff to intervene and keep the two apart. It was not just the nursing staff who tried to separate them. Some of the other residents were jealous, and Bob and Dorothy were forced to sneak around in order to continue their relationship.

Eventually, Bob's son moved him from the facility. Dorothy, who had blossomed under Bob's attention, lost more than 20 pounds and spent her days sitting near a win-

The section Dealing with Loss was contributed by Stephanie Gfeller, M.S., Research Assistant, Center on Aging, Kansas State University.

dow waiting for him to return. In one of her more lucid moments she asked her daugh-ter, a lawyer, to publicize the incident. The daughter asked if Dorothy could meet with Bob one last time to say goodbye. When Bob's family said no, she tried to make it hap-pen legally but was told that she could not make a case against the family because Bob could not be put on the witness stand because of his dementia. (Henneberger, 2008)

———————————————

Very little research has examined the effect of family members on older adult sex-uality, and yet family may be the primary influencing factor on how long-term care organizations approach sexual expression within their homes. Caregivers may ask family members about their loved one's morals or beliefs if the resident is un-able to speak for him- or herself. Family members may also share social histories that determine the types of relationships that caregivers steer residents into or away from. In addition, the family's reaction to their loved one's behavior may in-fluence the way the care home intervenes (Sidebar 4.1; Activity 4.1).

Many issues arise from family influences on resident sexuality, including sup-port and guidance for the noninstitutionalized spouse, adult children's reactions to a parent engaging in sexual expression or activity, and how to advocate for resident sexuality in the face of family resistance, each of which will be discussed in this chapter.

> Most of us have grown up not wanting to believe that our grandparents ever had sex, let alone that they might still be having it.

FAMILY INVOLVEMENT IN LONG-TERM CARE

A persistent myth exists that Americans abandon their older family members to nursing homes and assisted living. In truth, although Americans make use of res-idential living for older loved ones more frequently than families in other coun-tries, they hardly abandon them, visiting them often and sharing in their care at the facility. The emotions associated with seeking long-term care have much to do with how loved ones' sexual expression is accepted or resisted in these homes.

In a marital relationship, as one of the spouses becomes more incapacitated—either mentally or physically—the well spouse must assume some of the roles of the affected partner. This can cause fear, anger, resentment, and frustration. These emotions, coupled with the normal developmental difficulties of aging, create a recipe for stress.

Sidebar 4.1
Kansas State University Center on Aging Research

Research on resident sexuality indicates a wide range of family reactions to sexual expression in a nursing home setting (Doll, Bolender, & Hoffman, 2011). The Kansas State University Center on Aging asked a group of Kansas nursing home administrators and social workers to characterize family responses to resident sexuality. As indicated by the chart below, these range from supportive to embarrassed. (Study participants were allowed to check more than one response in light of the possibility of multiple instances of sexual expression in the home.) Most (60%) felt that family members had been supportive of facility actions when a loved one had expressed him- or herself sexually, and 40% had been indifferent or really did not care what happened. But 25% of the respondents said that family members would be unsupportive of any sexual activity or intimacy on the part of their loved one. Fewer were angry, but many were embarrassed by the actions of their loved one. One wrote that the family members had been "humiliated" by their mother's actions.

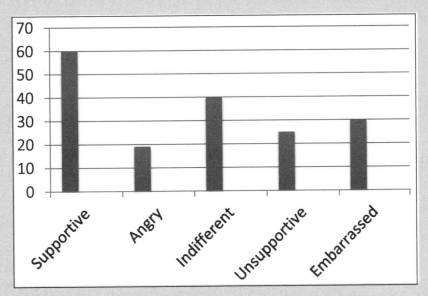

Sidebar 4.1 figure. Family reaction to sexuality in nursing homes by percentage

Caregiving spouses must also adjust their expectations of their loved one, as the cognitive or physical losses affect nearly every aspect of a marital relationship. The key to a successful adjustment is the ability to let go of old expectations. If the caregiver spouse succeeds, the affected spouse does not feel the pressure to live up to old expectations. This process, however, can be long and sorrowful.

The well spouse who is forced to seek formal caregiving for the affected spouse (especially placement in a long-term care home) experiences another uncomfortable wave of emotions, perhaps relief tinged with guilt, sorrow, disappointment, and grief. When the placement begins, the caregiver spouse may try to maintain active involvement in their loved one's care in the nursing or assisted living home. Family members may believe that sharing in their relative's care is a highly regarded personal goal. Staff members should be sensitive to these feelings and do what they can to guide the caregiver spouse in accepting the situation.

Adult children experience similar issues as they find themselves in a role reversal—parenting their parent. Assuming more and more responsibility in caring for an aging parent occurs at a time when many adult children are dealing with the stresses of raising children, establishing careers, preparing for retirement, and facing their own fears of aging.

Aging people do not come with instruction manuals. Spouses or adult children, cast in the role of caregiver, struggle with how much or how little to do for their aging spouse or parent. The results of doing too much can be as devastating as doing too little. Doing too much can lead to learned helplessness and greater dependence. Psychologically, doing too much sends the message that the older adult is incapable or incompetent, a perception that he or she quickly accepts (internalizes) and acts upon. Older individuals can become incapable of doing things for themselves very quickly when they stop believing that they are competent. One study found that when older adults who were capable of moving around on their own moved into a nursing home, they needed help getting out of a chair within 2 weeks (Pawlson, Goodwin, & Keith, 1986).

The loss of function that comes from learned helplessness may be more disabling than the diseases that can affect mobility, decision making, and the ability to perform basic tasks. The psychological effects of learned helplessness are pervasive, affecting older adults' beliefs in their ability to function not only physically, but also psychologically and socially. It can even cause older adults to question their ability to maintain intimate relationships. Beliefs about competency have a significant effect on sexuality. On the one hand it may lead to older individuals suppressing sexual feelings because they believe themselves incapable of meeting their own needs, and on the other they may express themselves in inappropriate sexual ways in an effort to demonstrate some control and competency.

Sometimes staff caregivers do too much for certain residents out of love and compassion, but this can also occur because it saves time. It can take a lot of patience to allow an older adult to perform activities of daily living at his or her own pace. Caregivers may not recognize that their own loving care or assistance in the interest of saving time can undermine an older adult's level of competence.

> I once met with a group of family members to explain the changes in culture that were happening in the home that their loved one was living in. I described new schedules and new environmental designs and highlighted that residents were now given the opportunity to make many more decisions regarding their care. One wife threw up her hands and said in disgust, "If you gave my husband the choice, he would never take a bath. The next thing I know I'm going to drive up to the place and he'll be out playing in the street!"

It is hard for many family members to surrender the need to control, and they may challenge the staff members who suggest that they know more than family about how to care for a loved one. These challenges may become more apparent in issues as polarizing as sexual expression.

Dealing with Loss

It is critical for staff to recognize the feelings that family members experience when moving a loved one to a long-term care home. Such recognition is necessary for healthy transitions and for establishing a trusting relationship between the family and the caregivers. This relationship will lead to more successful teamwork toward developing a holistic care plan, which should include intimacy and sexuality.

Placing a loved one in a home is a loss that must be grieved in much the same way that people grieve death. Kübler-Ross (1997) defined five stages of dealing with a loss—denial, anger, bargaining, depression, and acceptance. Not everyone goes through all of these stages, and they do not necessarily go through them in a specific order.

Denial

Denial is a state of shock, and individuals recover from it gradually. A family member may not really want to believe that a loved one has changed or is failing in health and instead might choose to believe that this is only a temporary state and that everything will return to normal soon.

> A man recently placed his wife in a nursing home. Although he wanted to keep her home, he realized he could not. Once she was admitted he did not come back to visit her for days at a time. The rest of the family could not understand his behavior as he had always been close to his wife. The daughter decided to ask her dad why he was not visiting at the home, and he replied, "I know she is there, but if I do not go see her I can pretend she is somewhere else."

When a family member reacts in such a way, it may remove an important support and intimate relationship from the new resident, who may react by seeking other meaningful relationships in the home. It is possible that the resident may also be feeling denial ("This is only temporary. I'll be going home soon."). In this case, the resident may fail to make meaningful connections in the long-term care facility.

Anger

The caregiving spouse or family member may experience feelings of anger for having let a loved one down by moving him or her to a home. Nursing home staff frequently see this in family members. Often this anger is misplaced and directed toward the caregivers at the home.

> Mary promised her husband she would never put him in a nursing home. He had always wanted to die on the farm. After a stroke left him partially paralyzed she had to admit that she could not care for him at home. After Ed moved to the home, Mary visited at least once a day. During each visit she would always find something wrong with the care he was receiving. Even when everything was being done to ensure Ed's needs were all being fulfilled, she still found something to complain about. She did not seem to understand she was upset with herself for breaking a promise to Ed. Instead of finding a way to deal with the broken promise, she pushed her feelings off onto the staff.

A spouse or other family member who is in the anger stage may be blinded to the benefits that the resident may receive from new loving relationships. Being unable to think clearly about the situation, a family member may respond out of anger and not good sense.

Bargaining

In this stage a family member may be tempted to make deals to ensure that a loved one's care needs are met. These deals might be with God (Please, God, I'll go to church every Sunday if you make my father well so I can take him home.), with the resident, with another family member, or with staff.

> When asked how a family member knew that her mother was receiving good care at the home, she said, "Each time I go to visit mother, I take some candy or cookies for her room. I like to let the staff know that it is there and that I want them to have it. I think they take better care of her when they know they are getting something in return."

Depression

When placing a loved one in long-term care, some family members may experience some emotional or physical changes, such as decreased energy, changes in sleep patterns or eating habits, loss of interest in normal activities, feelings of hopelessness, a persistent sad mood, irritability, or excessive crying. Such changes may indicate depression, and these people should consider seeing their doctor.

> Staff members noticed that Mary Jean had changed since she'd first come to visit her mother at the home. She had lost weight, she seemed to have no energy, and her bubbly personality had gone. Two of the nurse assistants were worried about her, and they visited with the social worker to see if she would talk to Mary Jean about seeing a doctor.

Family members who are depressed will have a hard time providing much support to the resident. In fact, the resident may feel the need to help the family member and may not be able to concentrate on his or her own needs. If the relationship had been sexual, it is likely that the depression will hinder the ability to be intimate, creating yet another loss for the resident.

Acceptance

Upon realizing that the placement was for the best, the family caregiver reaches acceptance, which can frequently coincide with the acceptance felt by the resident.

> Before my father came here he lived with me. It was so humiliating for him when I had to change his wet clothes. Now when I visit, I can talk to him like I used to. I can ask his advice and he can look me in the eye again.

The relief that comes with the acceptance stage may open the door for the return of intimacy. Many spouses report renewed affection for loved ones when they reach this stage. At this stage staff may need to begin to think about how they can provide privacy for the couple. (To learn more about what it feels like to experience loss, see Activity 4.2.)

The decision to place a loved one in a nursing home is fraught with guilt and pain. Much of the anger and criticism family members may direct toward staff and nursing home administration is a coping mechanism, possibly a way for them to continue to see themselves in the caregiver role. This need to control can continue for quite some time after the resident's admittance to the home. When a sexual situation arises, family caregivers may feel a renewed sense of loss of control in trying to deal with the situation.

One way for staff to help alleviate the guilt and loss spouses feel when their mate moves to a care facility is to do everything possible to make the spouse feel welcome in the facility. One continuing care retirement community in Kansas had overbuilt assisted living units. They decided to open one wing for residents with Alzheimer's disease and to allow spouses to co-reside for a relatively low fee.

Staff should assure visiting spouses that they will be afforded privacy. This may be achieved by allowing locked doors, posting do-not-disturb signs, and making special arrangements for conjugal visits. One of the easiest ways to promote privacy is to make certain that staff wait for permission to enter after knocking on a door.

SPOUSAL ISSUES WITH SEXUALITY

Sexuality can pose complex issues for well spouses. Caregiver spouses may find that they cannot separate their role of providing care to their loved from their role as a sexual partner to their affected spouse. Any type of chronic disease can intensify a marriage's strengths or weaknesses that may have existed before the onset of the disease. A partner may be so changed by disease that the attributes that once were physically attractive are lost. He or she may also exhibit behaviors that are not conducive to sex or sexual attraction, such as poor hygiene, self-absorbed behavior, incontinence, and communication problems. Female caregivers in particular may feel that the sexual attention offered or forced on them by a spouse with dementia is neither love or a way to meet the caregiver spouses's needs. Engaging in sexual activity with an affected spouse may be seen as a cost of the relationship rather than a reward or an exchange of love.

In one study (Duffy, 1995), hypersexual interest displayed by male spouses caused their caregiver wives to have feelings ranging from mild irritation to strong aversion. However, male caregivers in the same study did not have any complaints about their wives' increased receptiveness to sexual overtures.

When spouses must make decisions regarding sexual activity they may ask these questions:

- How am I obligated as a spouse to a husband or wife who no longer recognizes me?
- How do I maintain a sexual relationship when my feelings toward my spouse have changed?
- How do I handle the feelings of anger, frustration, and entrapment?
- How do I cope with my spouse's changes in sexuality (suspicion, hypersexuality, accusations of unfaithfulness)?
- How can I meet my spouse's needs? I love my spouse, but I cannot bring myself to be intimate with him/her? (See Sidebar 4.2.)

Moving a spouse to a care home can actually increase affection between partners. In community-dwelling older couples, affection increases with age, and interest in sexuality remains high; however, frequency of intercourse declines. In one study, researchers found that affection increased dramatically in spousal pairs when an affected spouse was moved to a nursing home (Kaplan, 1996). The authors surmised that the alleviation of stress in the caregiving spouse caused a renewal of affection between the two spouses. Many spouses visit the nursing home almost daily and provide care for their mate during visits. These caregivers may be experiencing a re-emergence of their previous feelings for their loved one.

SPOUSAL SHARED ROOMS

Most nursing home policies make provisions for married people to share a room in the nursing home or assisted living residence. These policies, however, have caveats about medical contraindications or other "reasonable" limits to consensual sexual activity. In other words, a medical director may determine that married couples should not live together in the nursing home if it may be physically or medically harmful to do so. Few institutions have been able to provide a shared room when one spouse has greater care needs than the other, and frequently one may live in assisted living while the other resides in skilled nursing care (Activity 4.3).

Sidebar 4.2
Celibacy?

A sex educator, Peggy Brick, presented sexual information to a retirement community. She asked residents to write down their questions or concerns. One of the questions, asked by more than one person, was, "Must I be celibate if my spouse is no longer interested in sex?" While this question may have been asked by someone who is still living with a spouse, it could also arise when one spouse can no longer live at home. Is it possible to maintain a commitment as spouses when one lives in long-term care while the other engages in an extramarital relationship?

CBS Sunday Morning aired a story about two reporters, how they met, married, and traveled the world until she was diagnosed with early-onset Alzheimer's disease while still in her 40s. He tried caring for her in their home, but ultimately had to move her into assisted living. Gradually she could no longer remember who he was, other than a kind stranger who made her smile. As he experienced the "loss" of his spouse, he eventually began a relationship with someone else. Now he and his new partner together visit his wife in the long-term care home.

Some of us may think of this as a strange scenario, and it is easy to imagine that some long-term care personnel may have a hard time accepting this situation for religious or moral reasons. In the television segment, however, the wife clearly benefits from having both Mr. Happy, as she now calls her husband, and his friend visit regularly.

This situation likely would not often be the case. Some spouses become involved in another relationship and gradually decrease their visits to the nursing home or assisted living facility. The resident may experiences this as a loss, something staff must recognize and assist the resident in dealing with.

Phyllis and George had been married for 68 years when they moved to a nursing home. Their children were adamant that their parents would share a room in the home. Several weeks later when one of the state regulators was visiting in the building, she noticed bandages on Phyllis's arms and legs. When the state regulator inquired about them she was told that George had been "a little rough" the night before. Further investigation revealed that he had been abusing his wife for as long as anyone could remember. When the administrator was asked why the couple was in the same room, he responded that the children were insistent that they live together to save expenses. The regulator, fearful for Phyllis's well-being, ordered her to be removed from the room she shared with George. Phyllis did not want to live with anyone else, and 3 weeks later she was still complaining about the move.

This scenario is rare. In most situations where spouses share a room the outcomes are very good. Being together maintains continuity and can provide a sense of security when a resident is experiencing many stressful changes. Staff can make special accommodations for married couples (moving beds together or allowing them to bring a bed from home). Couples may also be given two adjoining rooms, using one for a bedroom and the other for a living room for receiving guests and watching television.

The needs of both residents, however, should be carefully considered before allowing spouses to move into the same room. The challenge of moving from a living environment of a large house and community to a single room can create special adjustment problems for the couple. It may not always be appropriate for a married couple to share the same room.

I once visited a home where the staff bragged about the "cute little couple" in room 24B. They had been married for more than 70 years, and everyone thought it was very special that they could be together there at the home. As I sat in the atrium the husband came and sat down beside me. From our conversation I got the distinct impression that the current living arrangement was not comfortable for him—this was a bit too much closeness. He indicated that he took every opportunity he could to get out of the room.

While older married residents are encouraged to share rooms, couples who are not married may find it difficult to assert those same rights. This may be especially true of same-sex couples. The fear of being "caught" is enough to discourage residents from sexual activity, especially for lesbian, gay, bisexual, and transgender residents (see Chapter 7).

FAMILY FEELINGS ABOUT RESIDENT SEXUALITY

Families have an enormous impact on residents' sexuality. This happens even before a resident moves into a care facility. Adult children can influence their parents' sexuality by believing that old age signals decreased sexual interest, and may incorporate that belief into caring for their parents. Over time, the parents may learn to accept this notion and live up to it, sort of a self-fulfilling prophecy. It has been suggested that children's negative attitudes about late life sexuality may be due, at least in part, to a subconscious belief that we reap what we sow. Parents may present sexuality to their children within socially proscribed parameters, and when those children become adults they apply those limits to their own aging parents.

Adult children as caregivers to their own parents may develop paternal attitudes. This is especially true when a parent has dementia and becomes more child-like and in need of protection. An adult child caregiver may view a sexual situation involving an aging parent as they would a pre-teen in a sexual situation (i.e., as unable to make an informed decision). The adult child feels it is important to make the decision for the parent.

Although families share with care staff their loved one's likes and interests prior to moving a parent into a facility, staff typically do not ask for and families do not provide details related to the parent's sexuality. It is likely that adult children of older residents seldom think about their parent's sexual needs. If they were asked, they would almost certainly assume that their parent's values regarding sexuality matched their own. Because sexuality is a taboo subject between generations, especially with one's own parent, it seems unlikely that younger people could have an accurate understanding of a parent's or grandparent's desires.

Family responses to a loved one engaging in sexual expression or activity with another resident in the long-term care home can range from asking staff to move their loved one or the other resident to another floor to instructing staff not to allow the physical relationship to accepting and even appreciating the benefits that are afforded their loved one from the new experience. Some adult children may feel jealous that their parent's affections are centered on someone else. They may also resent that their parent is not being loyal to a deceased parent. Financial concerns may also come into play. Going back to the case study at the beginning of the chapter, it turned out that Dorothy's family believed that Bob's son was concerned that Dorothy was a "gold-digger" seeking to take advantage of Bob and getting him to leave his money to her. Dorothy's family even suggested a prenuptial agreement in an effort to get Bob's son to consent to Bob and Dorothy's romance, but it did not alleviate his fears.

Nursing homes feel an obligation to tell family members about any sexual expression on the part of residents. In our own survey of 90 nursing home administrators we found that 40% would notify the family even if both residents involved in a relationship were capable of consenting. Regulations state that family or a designated guardian has to be notified about any major status change, and nursing homes fear repercussions from family and state regulating agencies. Some of the administrators in our study hated doing this ("Change the regulations and I won't tell!").

> I was recently told that a woman who frequently visited her 97-year-old aunt at a local nursing home was greeted one day by staff before she barely got in the door. They wanted her to know that Hilda had a "boyfriend." They appeared to be worried about how my friend would react to the news, especially since the boyfriend has a living wife.

Staff in a long-term care environment may be so attuned to the possibility of adverse consequences to residents sexually expressing themselves that they anticipate problems. They may wish to prevent these problems by sharing with family members information that in another environment would be held confidential (Activity 4.4).

SUMMARY

Families are very involved in the sexuality of residents in long-term care situations. In many cases, the organizations that care for residents will choose the direction of family members over the expressed desires of those residents. Long-term care facilities can support families with counseling and education. Some homes have found that with counseling most families accept their relatives' sexual activity.

Melinda Henneberger, whose story of Bob and Dorothy is shared at the beginning of the chapter, suggested that perhaps people should draw up a sexual power of attorney, because without one families will feel free to control the intimate lives of loved ones with dementia. This may sound extreme, but it does draw attention to a very serious problem.

REFERENCES

Doll, G., Bolender, B., & Hoffman, H. (2011). Sexuality in nursing homes: Practice and policy. Manuscript submitted for publication.

Duffy, L. (1995), Sexual behavior and marital intimacy in Alzheimer's couples: A family theory perspective. *Sexuality and Disability, 13*(3), 239–254.

Henneberger, M. (2008). An affair to remember. *Slate.* Retrieved from www.slate.com/id/2192178/.

Kaplan, L. (1996). Sexual and institutional issues when one spouse resides in the community and the other lives in the nursing home. *Sexuality and Disability, 14*(4), 281–293.

Kübler-Ross, E. (1997). *On death and dying.* New York: Scribner Classics.

Pawlson, L. G., Goodwin, M., & Keith, K. (1986). Wheelchair use by ambulatory nursing home residents. *Journal of the American Geriatrics Society, 34,* 860–864.

Planning for Family Reactions

Create a plan for how you would address each of the family reactions in the figure on page 79 (supportive, angry, indifferent, unsupportive, and embarrassed).

Experiencing Loss

Prior to the training session copy the cube pattern on the next page onto heavy paper and follow the instructions to make one cube, or die, for each small group. Divide a large training group into smaller groups of four to six people. Each person should take a piece of paper and write these five labels, numbering to five after each word: people, places, skills or abilities, things, activities. Next, ask the participants to list five people, places, and so on that are very important to them.

Each group will take turns rolling the die. If it lands on "things," the person rolling will have to cross off one of the important items from his or her list. If the die lands on the empty space, the player gets a pass. This is meant to simulate the feelings of loss one might experience when something important is taken away. Continue passing the die and removing items from the lists for about 10 minutes.

Ask the participants to describe how they were feeling as they played this game. Did they experience Kübler-Ross's stages of loss? Have them imagine how residents might feel upon admission to a nursing home. What losses would they experience and how might they be processing those losses? What about family members? How would loss affect the sexual life of a resident or a resident's loved one?

Instructions: Print the pattern on heavy paper. Cut out and fold with words on the outside. Glue tabs to create a cube.

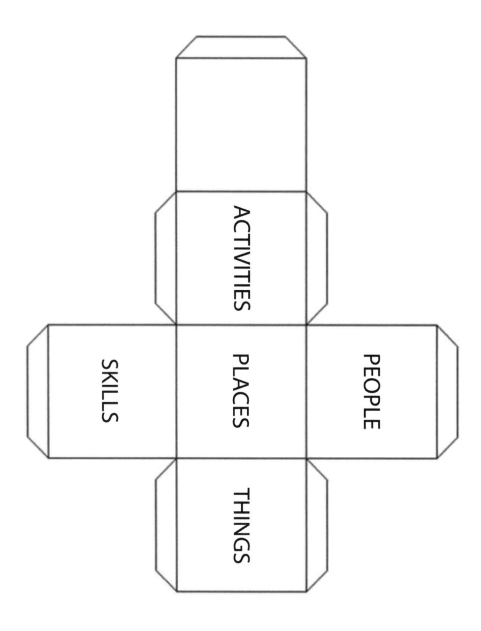

Discussion

Use the case studies provided in this chapter to lead a discussion. What is the facility's policy about shared rooms? What special accommodations are made for married couples living in the home? Can they share a room if they have different levels of care (e.g., he requires assisted living and she requires more skilled care)?

Role Playing

Role play the interactions among the specified parties in the following scenarios:

Scenario 1 roles:

Family member
Staff member (certified nursing assistant)

A resident (Ethel) has lived in the home for 3 weeks. She has developed an attachment to Charlie, another resident. On two occasions, when a family member has come to visit, Ethel has been found in Charlie's room. So far they seem only to be holding hands. The family member approaches the nursing assistant and wants to know what the staff will do to prevent this relationship from progressing.

Scenario 2 roles:

Ombudsman
Family member
Nursing home or assisted living administrator
Staff caregiver

The ombudsman has been notified by a family member that she feels the long-term care facility administration and staff are not doing enough to protect her loved one. In the past 6 months the staff have reported to the family member that they have found men in Joan's bed several times. The family is mortified by the situation, not just that she is having sexual relations, but also that she is seeing more than one man. They

Sexuality and Long-Term Care: Understanding and Supporting the Needs of Older Adults, by Gayle Appel Doll (Copyright 2012, by Health Professions Press, Inc.)

know that this behavior is out of character for Joan, who has always lived by high moral standards. They worry about the disgrace it will bring to their family if word spreads to the community. They are also upset by Joan's disloyalty to her former husband, and are concerned about the possibility of sexually transmitted diseases.

Dementia

OBJECTIVES

- Provide background information on types and effects of dementia
- List benefits of sexuality for people with dementia
- Examine consent issues
- Analyze "adultery" in the nursing home
- Review staff and family strategies

onna, a nurse at an assisted living dementia unit, discovered 69-year-old Eunice performing oral sex on 80-year-old Raymond. Donna ordered Raymond to pull up his pants and he yelled at her, telling her to get out of his room. Donna rushed off to find her supervisor. The nurse documented Raymond's behavior as "agitated" and filed a report with the state.

In the investigation that followed it became clear that Raymond and Eunice believed that they were married, even though Raymond's wife was still living and visited frequently. When Raymond's wife heard about the incident, she requested that staff keep the couple apart by any means, including physical or chemical restraints. The staff had concerns of their own; believing that Eunice was too cognitively impaired to consent to sexual relations, they felt a need to protect her. They believed Raymond posed a threat to Eunice's personal rights.

The care staff began using behavioral therapy with Raymond, repeatedly showing him pictures of his wife to reinforce that she—not Eunice—was his true wife. In addition, they placed him on an antipsychotic drug and tranquilizer for his agitation and on another medication intended to reduce his "disinhibited" behaviors. Despite these therapies he continued to be devoted to Eunice, and it was decided that they needed to be permanently separated.

Eunice became withdrawn and combative and was consequently prescribed a tranquilizer. Raymond started making overtures to other women, but neither he nor Eunice formed relationships with others like the one they had shared. (Adapted from McClean, 1994)

WHAT IS DEMENTIA?

The medical definition of dementia is *significant cognitive loss, severe enough to cause problems with occupational or social functioning; manifests in impairment of attention, memory, language, motor skills, orientation, judgment, and functional ability.* The prevalence of dementia is 14% in the over-70 population (Plassman et al., 2007). The frequency of dementia doubles every 5 years after the age of 60, with some researchers conservatively reporting that close to 40% of people who reach the age of 90 will have some form of cognitive loss great enough to be diagnosed as some form of dementia (Plassman et al., 2007).

Table 5.1 describes types of dementia and their known effects on sexuality in older adults. Alzheimer's disease (AD) is the most prevalent form of dementia, accounting for more than 60% of all cases. The disease is typically portrayed as having three stages—mild, moderate, and severe. During the early stage, people have trouble finding the right words or remembering names, lose or misplace objects, and begin to experience performance issues in social or work settings as well as a decline in the ability to plan and organize. In the moderate stage, individuals struggle with recalling recent events, have a reduced memory of personal history, and will begin to require assistance with the activities of daily living (ADLs), including dressing, bathing, and toileting. People with severe AD frequently lose their capacity for recognizable speech, need extensive assistance with ADLs, and gradually lose the ability to smile, hold their head up, walk without assistance, or sit without support.

> Intimacy and sexuality can be overlooked when considering the well-being of residents with dementia. The rights of privacy and intimacy may be denied to persons who cannot fight for them.

Sexual interest is usually nonexistent in the severe stage of AD. In the earlier stages sexual expression will vary among individuals. Most often individuals will retain patterns of sexual desire repeated throughout their life span; however, some may have an increased interest, perhaps as a way to maintain continuity with past behaviors or to demonstrate mastery of some area of their life.

Table 5.1 Types of dementia and their known effects

Type of Dementia	Description	Effect on Sexuality
Alzheimer's disease	The most common form of dementia. Caused by plaques and tangles in the brain.	Mixed, although usually resulting in apathy at later stages.
Vascular	Caused by poor blood flow to the brain possibly because of a stroke, diabetes, and hypertension.	Usually results in apathy.
Mixed	May be a combination of types of dementia such as Alzheimer's disease and vascular dementia.	Unknown
Dementia with Lewy bodies	Caused by abnormal protein deposits in nerve cells in the brain stem.	Unknown
Parkinson's disease	May not always result in dementia. Characterized by tremors, muscle tightness, and speech problems.	Usually results in apathy, but the medications may cause hypersexuality.
Frontotemporal	Pick's disease is the most prevalent. Damage to brain cells in the frontal and temporal lobes. Causes decline in social skills and emotional apathy.	May cause hypersexuality
Creutzfeldt-Jakob disease	Caused by a virus and spreads very rapidly. It is very rare.	Unknown
Normal pressure hydrocephalus	Appears to be caused by an accumulation of cerebrospinal fluid in the brain's cavities.	Unknown
Huntington's disease	An inherited progressive dementia, it causes memory problems, impaired judgment, mood swings, depression, and speech problems.	Some people feel a lack of will to live, and in some cases sexual disinhibition is demonstrated.
Wernicke-Korsakoff Syndrome	Caused by deficiency in vitamin B1, which often occurs in alcoholics but is also as a result of malnutrition, cancer that has spread throughout the body, or abnormally high thyroid hormone levels.	Unknown

The well spouse may experience a decrease in sexual attraction when the spouse with AD requires assistance with intimate activities such as bathing and toileting. There seem to be gender differences in attraction. Researchers have found that female caregivers are uncomfortable if their partner's interest in sex is heightened, whereas male caregiver spouses do not experience the same discomfort

(Duffy, 1995). They appreciate their wife's increased affection and interest in sex after the onset of the disease. Caregiver spouses report a change in the perceived relationship with their spouse as early as the end of the first stage of AD, when problems are serious enough to affect social and work performance (Activity 5.1).

Dementia and Sexual Interest

Several studies have indicated that interest in sexuality continues even when dementia is present (Kamel & Hajjar, 2004; Loue, 2005; Tabak & Shemesh-Kigli, 2006). As in populations of older adults without dementia, far fewer of these people are engaging in sexual activity than desire it. The need for intimacy appears to be something that lasts throughout the life span, but sexual interest and activity may diminish primarily due to the disabling effects of disease. Studies show varying interest and capability among residents with dementia, but most appear to be indifferent about sexual activity, especially in the later stages.

The memory of love is present even if one's memory is compromised.

THE EFFECTS OF DEMENTIA ON SPOUSAL CAREGIVERS

It may be helpful to caregivers to understand the effect that dementia may have had on a couple prior to a spouse with dementia moving into long-term care. This information can guide caregivers in developing a more empathetic approach with the resident as well as the spouse.

When one member of the couple is affected by dementia, expectations of mutuality and reciprocity are not fulfilled. Humans function in relationships by expecting equal rewards for the costs they commit. (If I invite you out to dinner it is with the expectation that you will do the same for me at a later date.) People who have dementia lose social conventions and do not remember to reciprocate. This can cause a great deal of tension between a couple when one spouse continues to give with no reciprocation.

It can be easy to forget the reasons for marriage if one of the partners is chronically forgetful, repeats the same questions constantly, experiences personality changes, and develops challenging behaviors. A spouse may feel alienated and withdraw affection that had been important to both partners. Financial concerns about the costs of caregiving may also undermine closeness and intimacy. These concerns can add to the chronic stress of caregiving.

Informal support networks may pull away when they are most needed. Families and friends do not take the vow "in sickness and in health" and sometimes withdraw from the couple due to their discomfort with the personality and other changes resulting from dementia. This loss of informal support networks can cause a spousal caregiver to feel disappointment and isolation.

The Sexual Life of an Older Couple When One Spouse Has Dementia

Kuhn (1994) found that the sexual life of a couple may be affected in a number of ways as the spouse with AD enters the early stages of disease. For instance, the spouse with AD may be sexually interested but have performance issues (impotency for the man, lack of vaginal lubrication or clitoral engorgement for the woman). These difficulties may lead to problems with self-esteem. In a couple with a previously strong relationship, the well spouse may be able to find ways to accommodate the changes. Alternatively, the well spouse may be ambivalent about making accommodations for sexual activity. Difficulties with performance may lead to avoidance or regulation of the frequency of sexual activity. The partner with AD may feel rejected, hurt, or angry.

In another scenario, the partner with AD may remain sexually interested and capable, which may be received well by the well spouse as a way to retain the continuity of at least one area of their life together. One happy man said that his wife was less inhibited with sex after she was diagnosed with Alzheimer's disease, and that she actually initiated it—something she had never done in the past. This degree of change in a spouse with AD, however, is not always well received by the well spouse. In some cases, the affected partner may become childlike. As the spouse with AD continues to lose functional ability, he or she may even lose the memory of lovemaking and any consideration of the spouse's sexual needs. Both partners may feel guilt and have trouble negotiating sex.

In a third scenario, the spouse with AD may become hypersexual. Some affected spouses may see sexual activity as a way to improve self-esteem and competency. The well spouse may not ask for help with this problem because of embarrassment. Sharing the issue may not get the support desired, especially if it is sought from a nonprofessional, such as a daughter or a friend.

Finally, the partner with AD may have no sexual interest or may think sexual activity is unacceptable based on a distorted self-perception of being too young or being unmarried. These individuals may believe their spouse is a stranger. Giving up sex may be acceptable to the well spouse, who may not have enjoyed it prior to the disease or who may feel repulsed by the changes in his or her spouse. There could be relief mixed with loss.

Research has found that affection frequently increases between spouses when the partner with AD is moved into long-term care (Kaplan, 1996). The relief of stress may produce more positive feelings from the caregiver spouse toward the mate. Caregivers may also be trying to make up for the guilt they feel about the placement.

Standard clinical practice would be to restore and promote sexual well-being for the couple experiencing AD. This, of course, may not be realistic given the privacy restrictions in long-term care. Restoring intimacy in other ways, however, should be a priority.

BENEFITS OF SEXUALITY AND INTIMACY FOR PEOPLE WITH DEMENTIA

Sexual expression is especially important in nursing homes because they are seen as places of isolation and loss, especially for residents with dementia. Physical contact is a beneficial means of communication, serving to calm and reassure. Sharing an intimate relationship can bring happiness, joy, and meaning to the life of an older adult who faces each day with confusion. Other emotions that sexual expression and intimacy can evoke include shared trust, warmth, humor, comfort, and safety. When residents are allowed to express themselves sexually caregivers have noticed decreases in mood disorders, behavioral disturbances, and excessive disability. Sexual expression and intimacy may also allow residents to feel more comfortable and at home in the long-term care setting and may improve their quality of life in physical, psychological, and spiritual terms.

> Sexual sensations are among the last of the pleasure-seeking biological processes to deteriorate and may provide an enduring source of gratification when few pleasures remain (Roach 2004).

ABILITY TO CONSENT

Long-term care homes typically rely on testing to determine cognitive ability, generally using the Mini-Mental State Examination (MMSE). This test can also be used to decide if a resident is capable of making decisions about sexual activity

(Activity 5.2). This objective test results in a score that can be used as a cutoff point in determining the ability to make decisions regarding one's well-being. The number 14 has been used by health care practitioners for consent for sexual activity. Care institutions usually operate under policies and rules that are derived from the organization's dependence on medical assessments. In other words, it is unusual to find homes that would use more subjective measures for determining consent.

For those who may not be familiar with the MMSE, an example of how one would be administered is given in Sidebar 5.1. An assessment such as the MMSE may be appropriate only for evaluating medical needs, not emotional ones, including whether a resident is able to consent to a sexual relationship. Relying solely on such an assessment ranks the resident's own desires below the needs of the family and the perceived needs of the nursing home or assisted living facility. These homes err on the side of caution because they are under intense pressure to avoid malpractice lawsuits and regulatory violations. Does this reliance on medical standards dehumanize and discriminate against people with dementia?

Everyone dealing with these issues struggles with identifying the authentic self after the onset of dementia. Is the authentic self the person who existed before the onset of the disease, or is it the new individual who is being shaped by the disease? Because nursing staff typically have no knowledge of who a resident was prior to the onset of dementia they are more likely to believe that the authentic self is the person they see before them in their care (Sidebar 5.2).

Interviewing to Assess Consent

Martin Lyden (2007) provides a detailed script for evaluating the right of people with disabilities to consent. The following procedure has been adapted for residents living in long-term care:

1. The person doing the assessment should have a comfortable relationship with the resident and should explain the purpose and the process of the assessment.

2. If the resident has impaired speech, someone who is familiar with and understands his or her speech pattern may be asked to assist. In some cases, family members may be invited to attend the session.

3. Begin the session by explaining

    "We are meeting today because you were referred by one of the staff members who believes that you might be interested in having a sexual relationship. Is this true?" If the answer is yes, continue with the

An Example of the Mini-Mental Status Exam (MMSE)

Maximum score is 30 points. People with Alzheimer's disease generally score 26 points or less, although this is not a test for Alzheimer's. A number of other causes can account for a low score.

SECTION 1: ORIENTATION (10 pts for giving the correct date and location)

Questions asked may include the following: What is the day of the week? What year was last year? What is the street name? What building are we in?

SECTION 2: MEMORY (PART 1).

Memorize three objects (e.g., car, apple, peanut). Repeating the three objects correctly scores a point for each word remembered. (3 points total)

    If the person fails to remember the three items, the person testing will repeat the words, but no points are given. The person taking the test will be told to remember the items because he or she will be asked to recall them later in the test.

SECTION 3: ATTENTION AND CALCULATION

This part of the test assesses the ability to concentrate on a tricky task. Two different types of tests are used, but only the best of the two scores will be included for the total score.

    Starting at 100, count backward by 7. One point is given for each correct subtraction with a maximum of 5 points. If this test does not go well, the person can be asked to spell a word, such as *lunch,* backward. (5 points possible)

SECTION 4: MEMORY (PART 2).

Recall the three items from Section 2. One point is given for each correctly recalled object.

Sidebar 5.1 (continued)

SECTION 5: LANGUAGE, WRITING, AND DRAWING

The person being assessed may be shown two everyday items, like a comb and a watch, and asked to name them. Sometimes this is done with picture cards. You score one point for each answer.

The next part is to repeat a tongue-twister sentence, such as "Pass the peas please." One point is given for repeating the sentence.

Next is a three-part process with instructions such as: Take this paper in your hand (1 point), fold it in half (1 point), place it on the floor (1 point). The instructions are given only once.

A card is then shown with a simple task written on it. The command may be "close your eyes." One point is given if the person does the task (e.g., closes his or her eyes).

The next step is to write a sentence on a piece of paper. If the sentence makes sense, one point is given.

Finally, the person is asked to copy a design of two intersecting shapes (see example below). One point is awarded for copying it correctly.

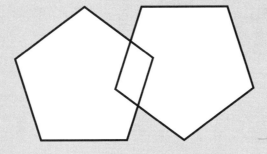

Source: Adapted from Kurlowicz & Wallace (1999).

interview. "I am meeting with you because it is important to determine if you have the capacity to have sexual relations with another person. Having capacity means that you have knowledge about sex and the consequences of that action. Would you like to have someone sit in with you during this meeting? I'll be asking you some questions about sex, relationships, and other things. You don't have

Sidebar 5.2
Dancing with Rose

In a very moving book titled *Dancing with Rose* published in 2007, author Lauren Kessler tells of her experience as a certified nursing assistant (CNA) in a dementia care unit. She trained to be a CNA following her own mother's death from Alzheimer's disease. Believing that she had failed her mother, she wanted to give back by working with older people who were experiencing the same challenges. She discovered a sense of relief from the guilt she had felt in choosing to move her mother to a home. She learned that family members see only the disease and what it has taken from their loved one and themselves. Professional care staff see these individuals as they are now, removing the pressure for them to try to remain who they once were. Staff members are more likely to see the humor, joy, love, and other personality attributes of persons with dementia that family members may miss due to their grief at the loss of their loved one's former self.

to know everything in order to be considered to have the capacity to have sex, so just do your best to give honest answers. When we are done with this meeting, I will write a report that will go to a small group of people made up of _____, _____, and _____ here at the home. Together, we will make a determination about whether you understand enough to have a sexual relationship. This group of people will keep your information confidential and will not share it with anyone except for the critical information your caregivers need to know. You will be told the group's decision."

4. There are three primary areas that are assessed: Rationality, knowledge, and voluntariness. Rationality is the resident's ability to evaluate the situation in order to make a knowledgeable decision. It may be assessed by examining the following: awareness of time, place, person, and event; ability to report events and to distinguish truth between fantasy and lies; ability to describe the process for deciding to have a sexual relationship and the ability to understand the verbal and nonverbal signals of another person's feelings.

In a knowledge assessment, residents should demonstrate an understanding of sexual activities and safe sex behaviors; the appropriate place and time for sexual activity; and awareness of another person's rights, including being able to honor their objection to the activity. Voluntariness means that the resident is able to take self-protective measures against unwanted advances.

An Example of a Consent Evaluation

Sidebar 5.3 presents a simplified version of an evaluation process that was created by clinical psychologist Peter Lichtenberg in 1997. It consists of a decision tree for determining a resident's competency to participate in a sexual relationship. Using this process, if a person's Mini-Mental score is less than 14, he or she would automatically be denied the opportunity to engage in an intimate relationship. Some would disagree with this form of assessment, preferring instead to use functional competency as a guide, which means that a person may be capable of performing in some areas while not in others and is a discrimination that the more global Mini-Mental assessment does not allow. Certainly, the MMSE does offer an objective measure that can make decisions regarding resident sexuality much less complicated.

If a resident is determined to be competent based on the Mini-Mental assessment, the next step is to determine the resident's ability to avoid exploitation. Does the resident have the ability to say no if he or she is uncomfortable with sexual contact? A second question may be to ask the resident if the sexual behavior is consistent with his or her previously held beliefs and values. The answer to this question will be subjective and may not be in the best interest of the resident's present needs (which is discussed further in the section later on substituted judgment). The intimate relationship would not be allowed if the resident were to express that the sexual activity goes against his or her previously held beliefs and values.

The next step is to determine the resident's level of awareness within the relationship. Is the resident aware of who is initiating the sexual contact? Does the resident believe the other person to be a spouse, or is the resident cognizant of the other's identity? Can the resident express what level of intimacy is comfortable? If the answers to these questions are yes, then the decision maker would move on to the next level. If the response is no, the resident would be denied the ability to have an intimate relationship.

Finally, the resident must be able to understand the risks involved in an intimate relationship. These may include the risk of contracting a sexually transmitted disease, but of utmost importance is the resident's ability to understand the consequences of a relationship that may be limited by circumstance and time (given that

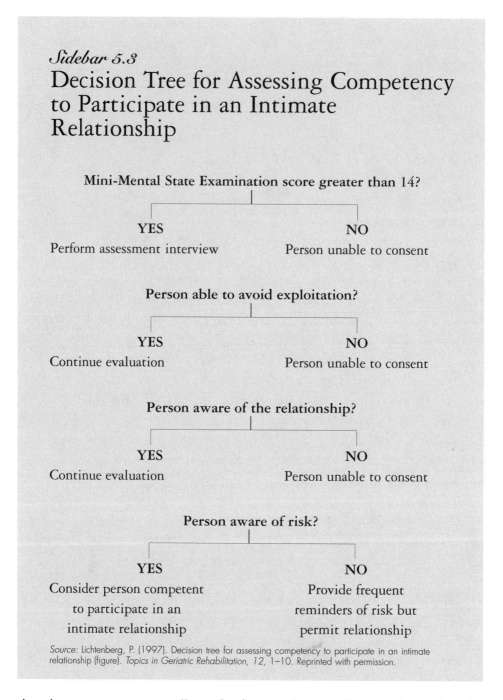

Sidebar 5.3

Decision Tree for Assessing Competency to Participate in an Intimate Relationship

Mini-Mental State Examination score greater than 14?

YES
Perform assessment interview

NO
Person unable to consent

Person able to avoid exploitation?

YES
Continue evaluation

NO
Person unable to consent

Person aware of the relationship?

YES
Continue evaluation

NO
Person unable to consent

Person aware of risk?

YES
Consider person competent
to participate in an
intimate relationship

NO
Provide frequent
reminders of risk but
permit relationship

Source: Lichtenberg, P. (1997). Decision tree for assessing competency to participate in an intimate relationship (figure). *Topics in Geriatric Rehabilitation, 12,* 1–10. Reprinted with permission.

the other person may eventually need to be moved or may die). Can the resident describe how he or she might react if the relationship should end (Sidebar 5.4)?

No matter how an organization chooses to go about determining consent, there are a few basic things to remember. The capacity to decide to have an intimate relationship should not be based on a one-size-fits-all concept. While some people affected by dementia will not be capable of handling their finances, they

Sidebar 5.4
Consent Literature from the Field of Developmental Disabilities

It may be instructive to review consent literature from outside the field of dementia. Consent is frequently debated for people with developmental disabilities. The following criteria, adapted from Ames and Samowitz (1995), have been suggested for inferring sexual capacity:

1. *Voluntariness.* A person must be able to voluntarily decide with whom he or she wants to have a sexual relationship. There should be no coercion.

2. *Safety.* Both participants should be reasonably protected from harm, such as the transmission of HIV or psychological harm (e.g., undesired separation).

3. *No exploitation.* A person should not be taken advantage of by a person with more power or status.

4. *No abuse.* There should be no abuse of a psychological or physical nature.

5. *Ability to say "no."* A person should be able to say "no" either verbally or nonverbally and to extricate him- or herself from an undesirable situation.

6. *Socially appropriate time and place.* Either the person should be able to choose the time and place appropriately or be willing to be directed toward that end.

might have very clear ideas about what they desire in a relationship. Cognitive memory may be affected while emotional memory is not. Feelings remain long after the "facts" have disappeared.

Dementia is an ever-changing disease state. Having determined capacity to consent to one relationship does not necessarily mean that the resident should be capable of having a relationship with another person. A second evaluation will be necessary to confirm that he or she has the capacity to consent in a different circumstance and time.

The more serious the risks or consequences of the sexual behavior or activity, the clearer the resident's decisional capacity needs to be. In many cases the home

"Bad" decisions made by residents with dementia do not necessarily indicate incompetence.

will make assumptions about the resident's ability to consent believing that the resident's ability to consent will be based on his or her previous values and goals, and so exercising consent will help the resident retain those values and goals. It is clear that these types of decisions require careful thought on the part of all stakeholders. Further, intrinsic to person-centered care is the expectation that a resident is included in these types of discussions, even if someone else is making decisions for him or her.

Problems with Consent Decisions

People with dementia living in long-term care are subject to higher levels of surveillance and regulation than are those who retain their cognitive ability. An incident of sexual expression can be viewed as a problem and a disruption of the social fabric of the environment. Sexual expression targeted at caregivers, sexual exploitation, public sexual expression, and any expressions that deviate from the heterosexual norm induce the greatest anxiety in caregivers.

While few people could object to the notion that people in long-term care living with dementia should have the same rights to sexual expression and intimacy as other residents, dementia complicates the issue. However beneficial it may be, resident sexual expression is a challenge for long-term care homes because residents may lack the legal capacity to consent to sex, and the consent they do give may be difficult to interpret. A resident with dementia might not be able to evaluate social situations rationally because of poor judgment, disorientation, and loss of memory. Because of these limitations it can be hard to determine if there is consent or abuse. For example, it could be deemed a criminal act if a woman with dementia thinks she is having sex with her husband when she is actually with another man in the home or if a resident with dementia does not understand a request to stop. It is a crime to engage in sexual conduct with an individual who is so mentally incapacitated that he or she cannot express consent. The courts rarely prosecute a mentally incapacitated individual who has sexual relations with a person who cannot consent because he or she does not meet the competency standards to stand trial. Despite the lack of prosecution, nursing home administrators and staff can come seriously close to criminally facilitating a sexual offense if they seem to encourage sex between individuals with dementia and it is hard to determine consent. If a family objects to their loved one engaging in sexual activity, facilities may also be held liable for the failure to protect a resident if a sexual encounter is deemed a physical assault. It is important that a long-term care facility have a consent policy regarding sexual expression for people with dementia and that staff members understand and abide by it. Activity 5.3 can be used to facilitate awareness of this critical issue.

THE DILEMMA OF "ADULTERY"

Perhaps the most severe family problems arise when a resident develops a sexual relationship in the long-term care home when he or she still has a living spouse. As already discussed, the administrative team must intervene to prevent unsafe and abusive relationships. What, however, should their involvement be when a resident with dementia, whose spouse lives elsewhere, engages in an intimate relationship with another resident?

Clear guidelines must exist to deal with these complex issues and should measure morals, the resident's prior values that were formed before the onset of dementia, and the resident's current well-being. The long-term care home might think that simply ending a relationship is the best course of action, but doing so may infringe on the resident's rights to privacy and autonomy.

Tenenbaum debated eloquently whether it is right to rely solely on the nonresident spouse's opinion when he or she objects to an adulterous relationship (Tenenbaum, 2009). Is the nursing home's highest obligation to the family member (spouse) or to the resident? Many spouses may believe that ending a relationship is what is best for the resident and would have been the decision the resident would have made had he or she been competent. Allowing the spouse to determine if the relationship continues may make sense when you consider that in 23 states, adultery is a crime. The standard definition of *adultery* is sexual intercourse between a married person and someone other than the person's spouse. It is unclear, however, if people with dementia who do not realize that they are married can commit adultery.

Some nursing homes fear prosecution as accomplices to the crime of adultery, but these fears are mostly academic because no one prosecutes adultery anymore. Public figures admit to it, and people may use it as grounds for divorce without worrying about their spouse being charged with adultery. In 1995, Justice Scalia questioned whether statutes against adultery were constitutional.

Tenenbaum argued that

> There is no reason to hold demented individuals to a higher standard than everyone else. Indeed, there may be less reason to prevent demented patients from committing adultery. Society's disapproval of extra-marital sex is based, in part, on the problems that may arise, such as "unplanned pregnancy, single parent families, di-

vorce, venereal disease and AIDS." Most of these concerns either do not apply to the elderly in nursing homes or are likely to be less of a problem. (p. 698).

While people with dementia may not be able to recall past events, they can still reproduce meaningful relationships by taking meaning from what they experience in the present, unrelated to personal history. This allows people with cognitive loss to live in the moment, creating a new self in relation to another person and restoring a sense of continuity.

The well-being of the resident should be the most important consideration for the nursing home. The Omnibus Budget Reconciliation Act of 1987 (OBRA) mandates that nursing homes "attain and maintain his or her highest practicable physical, mental and psychosocial well-being." With this goal in mind the nursing home should not take steps to end an intimate relationship based solely on the request of the nonresident spouse.

SURROGATE DECISION-MAKING APPROACHES

Faced with the necessity of developing guidelines and policies in response to this challenging dilemma when it arises in nursing homes, there are several different decision-making frameworks to consider using in finding a resolution and justifying the decision for all parties involved.

Substituted Judgment

Because the nursing home has an obligation to the well-being of the resident, the home would act as a surrogate decision maker for the married resident. This requires the nursing home to reach, as accurately as possible, the same decision that the married resident with dementia would reach if competent. This is referred to as *substituted judgment*. The care home would have to gather information about the resident's core values, philosophical and religious beliefs, morals, and patterns of behavior prior to the diagnosis of dementia. The courts like substituted judgment because it reflects the resident's own views and preferences.

Knowing that the resident would likely have respected the spousal relationship, the substituted judgment might be to end the adulterous relationship. Some character theorists would agree with this decision because they believe that we each create who we are by selecting core values that are stable over time. These values and how we live them make up our rational life plan. These same theorists recognize that we also have "brute" interests, which are sensations or feelings. Patients with dementia may lose their ability to reason and maintain their core values, but these theorists argue that the values we choose and nurture while we are rational should be respected over the brute desires that we may act upon when we are not competent.

The problem with this reasoning is that it is difficult for decision makers in a care home to accurately predict what the resident with dementia would have decided about an adulterous relationship if the individual were not cognitively affected by the disease. This is not likely to have been written into an advance directive, therefore the long-term care home would have to rely on the family to be surrogate decision makers. Some studies, however, have shown that family surrogates are often inaccurate in predicting what the patient would want (Houts, Smucker, Jacobson, Ditto & Danks, 2002; Kothari & Kirschner, 2007). This is probably caused by family members' emotional interests in believing that the loved one has values similar to their own, which is especially true in cases of adultery (Kayser-Jones & Kapp, 1989).

Nursing and assisted living homes have strong incentives to favor family views. The homes may be concerned about liability, and their staff realize that the community-living spouse can create more of a problem than the resident with dementia. Other family members will devalue the interests of the resident with dementia and defer to the well spouse to protect his or her feelings (Tenenbaum, 2009). ". . . the biases in the system favor relying on the opinion of the non-resident spouse" (Tenenbaum, 2009, p. 705).

Values and desires can change, so it does not always make sense to use a resident's history as a means of determining consent. It is impossible to predict the wishes of a person who becomes cognitively disabled. Also, some would say that an individual with dementia is no longer the person he or she once was. If there is disease or injury causing sufficient disruption in memory, the individual is no longer the same person (Sidebar 5.5). Respecting prior values may prevent the resident from having his or her present needs and desires met (Activity 5.4).

A number of years ago, a California physician learned that he had Alzheimer's disease. Believing that he did not want to live with that burden he asked his wife to have Dr. Kevorkian help him end his life when he reached a certain stage in his dementia. His wife agreed but when the time had come to call Dr. K. their son intervened, kidnapping his father and moving him to live with him in Michigan. The case ended in court. The son's argument was that his father was no longer the man that he was when he had requested to end his life. At this stage in his disease, he no longer remembered the reasons he did not wish to live and seemed to be living a happy and contented life. The court agreed.

Sidebar 5.5
Authentic or Precedent Autonomy

"The most popular way out of the nagging sense that the resident has been wronged is to rely on what medical ethicists call authentic or precedent autonomy. Every person to whom society grants such autonomy is assumed to possess an idealized moral agency. That agency is responsible for making decisions and for displaying a consistent pattern of habits and beliefs. The wishes and values of the "authentic moral self" are assumed to be fixed over time and across shifting contexts. Departures with one's past therefore become evidence of pathology; the misbehaving resident must, by the very act of misbehaving, no longer be capable of moral agency." (McClean, 1994, p. 38)

Best Interest

Best interest refers to what would benefit the resident the most and cause the least amount of harm. The resident's safety, health, and well-being are considered objectively, based on what a hypothetical average person would choose. No personal preferences are taken into account. The problem with using best interest is the difficulty in trying to remain objective. It is hard to avoid personal biases when one is acting as a substitute decision maker. Another problem is that best interest, because it makes assumptions about the resident, does not consider the resident's feelings and may rob him or her of the ability to choose (Activity 5.5).

> It is important that a long-term care facility have a consent policy regarding sexual expression for people with dementia and that staff members understand and abide by it.

Some experts believe that residents with dementia continue to maintain decision-making capacity into the later stages of the disease process (Mitty, 2007). In such a case it is important to be able to measure functional competence to assess whether a resident can make the decision to continue a so-called adulterous relationship. Functional competence means that a person may be incompetent in some areas but not others. This measurement maximizes residents' autonomy by allowing them to maintain control over some aspects of their life. Nursing homes are meant to provide care in a manner that is the least restrictive of independence and freedom.

There are four steps in determining functional competence (Tenenbaum, 2009):

1. Determine whether the resident has the ability to express his or her desires. They do not have to be expressed orally but can be communicated through a consistent pattern of behavior.

2. Determine what critical interests or values might be affected by acting on those desires. The resident should understand the consequences and implications of his or her decisions, especially important life values and goals that are affected. Family feelings, the importance of being remembered a certain way, and religion should all be considered.

3. Once these interests are identified the next step is to determine if the resident can adequately consider these interests in making the decision. A resident who can adequately understand the consequences of a decision should be considered functionally competent. If not, go to step 4.

4. The nursing or assisted living home needs to decide whether the value of the intimate relationship to the resident outweighs the value of the critical interests affected. Given the knowledge available about the benefits of intimacy to the resident, Tenenbaum believes that the relationship should be heavily favored (Tenenbaum, 2009).

Authentic Self

Some argue that the *authentic* self is the most significant consideration in determining consent for sexual activity. If the self prior to the onset of dementia is authentic, then previously held morals, values, and practices should guide the caregiver in the interventions regarding sexual activity. It may be deemed more important to protect the resident's dignity in preventing a resident from engaging in sexual activity that he or she would otherwise have found offensive than to allow any apparent enjoyment of the relationship. If, however, the present self is judged to be authentic, then the pleasure derived from the intimate relationship should take precedence. Because of the changes in personality caused by dementia, the present self may not re-

It would be difficult to create policies for the authentic self. Policies should be flexible enough that each case can be evaluated individually. There is no black-and-white solution to address the unique needs and protect the rights of residents with dementia and no case where only substituted judgment or only best interest should be considered.

semble the previous self at all. Staff may find that trying to direct the resident to behave as the person he or she was prior to dementia may cause anxiety and behavior problems. Despite these difficulties, in medical settings, substituted judgment, or the previous self, is generally the chosen decision-making model. Nursing home staff and administration as well as family members generally make the determination of which model to use.

STAFF RESPONSES TO SEXUAL EXPRESSION IN RESIDENTS WITH DEMENTIA

There is a range of long-term care responses to sexual expression, from forced celibacy to encouraging sexual relationships. Generally speaking, sexual expression in dementia care is seen as a disruption. The physical environment of the home is not conducive to intimate relationships. Also at issue is the need to balance the perspective of the individual resident with that of the wider resident body. There may be an influence of a resident subculture, especially when the home has a religious affiliation.

Some long-term care homes limit patients' opportunities for sexual gratification due to potential liability issues, burdens on staff, and concerns about family attitudes. Because of all of these challenges, many staff actively prevent sexual encounters through physical and psychological means. Long-term care service providers walk a fine line in terms of ethical principles. On the one hand they are pledged to provide safety, but on the other hand they risk denying residents their rights when they withhold sexual activity from residents with dementia. Our moral codes were not developed for people with cognitive loss. Residents deserve to have their situations examined compassionately and individually. Each case is different, and many residents may still retain the ability to make some decisions about relationships, at least in the early stages of their dementia.

The psychological means employed to control resident sexuality may include stifling sexual expression by showing disapproval or by threatening and punishing a resident. Other measures include moving a resident to another floor, denying the use of private space, using restraints, putting clothes on backward or dressing residents in zipperless jumpsuits, imposing curfews, and using nighttime nursing checks. Imposing any of these measures may deny residents

"As alien as some new behaviors may be to the family and friends of the residents, they can be understood as new possibilities, rather than pathologies, that might ease the terrors of the isolation and fragmentation of dementia." (McClean, 1994, p. 39)

Sidebar 5.6
The Effectiveness of Dementia Care Units

Staff and administrators must try to address individual needs and desires while attending to the rights of the resident population at large. People with dementia may exhibit disruptive behaviors, such as wandering, taking things from other residents' rooms, repetitive questions or vocalizations, and unwanted sexual behaviors. Many nursing homes have built dementia care units to better manage these undesired activities. Anecdotal evidence has been mixed on the quality-of-life outcomes for residents living in these units. They benefit from a safe environment and specialized programming that may help to eliminate their problem behaviors. Some of the best outcomes may be that these disruptive behaviors are out of sight and out of mind for residents who do not have dementia. Sometimes residents who wander into other rooms are interpreted as having sexual intent. Dementia care units may reduce the number of complaints about unwanted sexual expression because of the reduction in these incidents.

their rights (Sidebar 5.6). One strategy for averting potential problems is to include a resident's sexual history in admissions records, including sexual orientation, sleeping arrangements at home, and current level of sexual interest and capacity (see Chapter 6). Such knowledge raises the awareness of staff members to the needs of residents (Activity 5.6).

DISCUSSION

Return to the story at the beginning of the chapter. Nearly all the staff agreed that Eunice joined Raymond of her own accord and never exhibited resistance to his advances. They recognized that Eunice and Raymond seemed to enjoy each other's company. The other residents were undisturbed by the relationship.

Given what you know now from reading this chapter, how would you have counseled the key stakeholders in this incident?

SUMMARY

Sexuality and the need for sexual expression continue even when dementia is present. The benefits of sexual expression and intimacy can enhance the quality of life for people with AD and other forms of dementia. The most important strategy for long-term care staff and administrators regarding the sexuality of people with dementia is to formulate a policy for determining a resident's ability to consent. Input for the policy should come from all of the stakeholders, including residents, family members, staff, and administration. The policy should be flexible enough to address the unique needs and protect the rights of residents with dementia, not just speak to what is best for the organization.

Staff and family must find the balance between protecting vulnerable residents and allowing them the freedom to risk making good or bad choices. It may be hard to decide if the resident is fully competent, partially competent, or fully incompetent and unable to make decisions regarding intimate relationships. Many people think that residence in a nursing home or other care facility implies incompetence. But it is unlikely that anyone loses full capacity until the later stages of dementia, so an all-or-nothing approach may be inappropriate.

Residents with AD or other forms of dementia still need recognition, approval, affection, and acceptance, even though they may be unable to return affection and attention in any meaningful way. Family and staff should follow these assumptions, which are adapted from Ballard (1995):

1. Individuals with AD may behave in unpredictable, irrational, and childish ways. However, they will retain adult feelings and should not be treated like a child.

2. People with AD are still sexual and may express a variety of sexual behaviors. Emotional security, trust, self-esteem, and physical closeness are all important to how a person feels cared for and valued.

3. You cannot force someone with AD to remember. Many of the conventions, values, and beliefs about sex and sexual behavior may be forgotten.

4. Behaviors are not always what they seem. Individuals with AD may appear to be difficult or may express inappropriate behaviors as a result of feeling frustrated, frightened, or embarrassed. They may not understand the consequences of their behavior. What looks like an overture for sexual activity may be a request for affection, attention, or reassurance.

5. The resident will become more dependent over time, often while resisting assistance or being thoughtless or indifferent to you and your needs. You might be mistaken for someone else, and your actions may be misunderstood.

6. As the world of the AD resident becomes more confusing the key to controlling difficult behavior is to provide a secure and predictable environment. Keep changes to a minimum and offer reassurance. Hold hands, speak calmly, and offer soothing music.

7. People with AD respond to warmth, respect, and dignified treatment.

REFERENCES

Ames, T., & Samowitz, P. (1995). Inclusionary standard for determining sexual consent for individuals with developmental disabilities. *Mental Retardation, 4,* 264–268.

Ballard, E. (1995). Attitudes, myths, and realities: Helping families and professional caregivers cope with sexuality in the Alzheimer's patient. *Sexuality and Disability, 13*(3), 255–270.

Duffy, L. M. (1995). Sexual behavior and marital intimacy in Alzheimer's couples: A family theory perspective. *Sexuality and Disability, 13*(3). 239–254.

Houts, R., Smucker, W., Jacobsen, J., Ditto, P. & Danks, J. (2002). Predicting elderly outpatients' life-sustaining treatments over time: The majority rules. *Medical Decision Making 22,* 39–52.

Kamel, H. K., & Hajjar, R. R. (2004). Sexuality in the nursing home, part 2: Managing abnormal behavior—Legal and ethical issues. *Journal of the American Medical Association, 5,* S48–S52.

Kaplan, L. (1996). Sexual and institutional issues when one spouse resides in the community and the other lives in the nursing home. *Sexuality and Disability, 14*(4), 281–293.

Kayser-Jones, J. & Kapp, M. (1989). Advocacy for the mentally impaired elderly: A case study analysis. *American Journal of Law and Medicine, 14*(4), 353–376.

Kessler, L. (2007). *Dancing with Rose: Finding life in the land of Alzheimer's.* New York: Penguin Books.

Kothari, S. & Kirschner, K (2007). Decision-making capacity after TBI: Clinical assessment and ethical implications, in *Brain injury medicine: Principles and practice,* (Nathan D. Zaser, Ed.) New York: Demos Medical Publishing.

Kuhn, D. (1994). The changing face of sexual intimacy in Alzheimer's disease. *The American Journal of Alzheimer's Care and Related Disorders & Research,* Sept./Oct., 7–14.

Kurlowicz, L., & Wallace, M. (1999). The Mini-Mental State examination (MMSE). Best Practices in Nursing Care to Older Adults, 3. Retrieved from www.isu.edu/nursing/opd/geriatric/MMSE.pdf.

Lichtenberg, P. A. (1997). Clinical perspectives on sexual issues in nursing homes. *Topics in Geriatric Rehabilitation, 12,* 1–10.

Loue, S. (2005). Intimacy and institutionalized cognitive impaired elderly. *Care Management Journals, 6,* 185–190.

Lyden, M. (2007). Assessment of consent capacity. *Sexual Disabilities, 25,* 3–20.

McClean, A. (1994). What kind of love is this? *The Sciences, 34*(5), 36–39.

Mitty, E. (2007). Decision making and dementia. *Try this: Alzheimer's Association Best Practices,* D9. Chicago, IL: Alzheimer's Association.

Plassman, B., Langa, K., Fisher, G., Heeringa, S., Weir, D., Ofstedal, M., Burke, J., Hurd, M., Potter, G., Rodgers, W., Steffans, D., Willis, R. & Wallace, R. (2007). Prevalence of dementia in the United States: The aging, demographics and memory study. *Neuroepidemiology, 29,* 125–132.

Roach, S. (2004). Sexual behavior of nursing home residents: Staff perceptions and responses. *Journal of Advanced Nursing, 48,* 371–379.

Tabak, N., & Shemesh-Kigli, R. (2006). *The size and characteristics of the residential care population: Evidence from three national surveys.* Washington, DC: Office of the Assistant Secretary for Planning and Evaluation, U.S. Department of Health and Human Services.

Tenenbaum, E. (2009). To be or to exist: Standards for deciding whether dementia patients in nursing homes should engage in intimacy, sex and adultery. Albany Law School Research Paper No. 15. *Indiana Law Review, 42*(3). Retrieved from http://papers.ssrn.com/sol3/papers.cfm?abstract_id=1470316.

Understanding Dementia

This activity is meant to simulate the experience of dementia, specifically some of the confusion that residents with dementia may feel.

You will need a small hand mirror, a piece of paper, and something to write with for this activity. Hold the mirror in your nonwriting hand and place the paper on a table in front of you, pencil or pen in your hand in preparation to draw. Now position the mirror over your shoulder on the nonwriting side. Look into the mirror and move it until you can see the paper lying on the table. Now, looking only at the mirror and the reflection of the paper, draw a picture of a house. When you have completed that task, draw a clock with the hands placed at 10 minutes past 3:00.

When you have finished, take a few minutes to reflect on your feelings. Did you have an emotional response to the activity? Were you frustrated? Imagine feeling this way all the time.

To apply this activity to the discussion of sexuality in persons with dementia, consider how important it might be to retain some levels of mastery and control. Being able to continue to express oneself sexually may be one of the last remaining comforts of old age.

Sexuality and Long-Term Care: Understanding and Supporting the Needs of Older Adults, by Gayle Appel Doll (Copyright 2012, by Health Professions Press, Inc.)

Take the MMSE

Have a group of staff members take the Mini-Mental State Examination (MMSE). Divide the group into pairs. One person will administer the test to the other, and then the pair can reverse positions. Upon completion of the test, paired members can discuss with each other the assessment's effectiveness in determining who might be capable of making decisions about sexual activity. Why do you think that some long-term care organizations use this method to decide who might be able to provide consent?

Consent Policies

Search the Internet for consent policies. They may be easily found for the disabilities community but should also be available for geriatric populations. Make copies of the consent policies found and ask a small group to review them. What elements can everyone agree on? Compare these policies to your own organization's. Do you think that your policy for consent for sexual expression should be different from or the same as the policy for consent for other types of activities?

Substituted Judgment:
A Case Study

When Alice moved to the nursing home because of her dementia, her family reported that she had always been an early riser, "getting up with the chickens" to start her day. Based on this information the staff woke her every morning at 6:00 and gave her a cup of coffee and something to eat. Alice was cranky all day every day, which was a surprise to her family, who had known her to be sweet and loving. Finally, in desperation, her nursing home caregivers decided they would let Alice sleep as long as she wanted without waking her. Alice slept until 10:00, and when she woke her sunny disposition had returned.

Can you think of times when a person working with older residents with dementia should question life history? Have you done it yourself? Can you think of ways that residents are no longer the same person they once were? Are some of those changes positive? Have you shared the observation of changes with family?

If a resident with dementia is truly a changed person, then basing care decisions on his or her earlier values would be like having strangers make decisions for the person. Given this argument, some believe that basing care decisions on the best interests of the resident is better than using substituted judgment.

Best Interest

Staff members in nursing homes use best interest all the time, especially when it comes to diabetic diets. Let us imagine that Charlie, who is diabetic, would like to have a dessert every night (and he really cannot stand the no-sugar sweets his caregivers keep trying to give him). Work through the questions to determine if it is in Charlie's best interest to eat desserts.

1. Can Charlie tell you what he wants? How does he tell you? Are you sure he knows what he wants?

2. What critical interests or desires may be affected if his request is granted?

3. Is Charlie aware of the consequences of eating a dessert every night and is he capable of understanding what may happen?

4. If he is not capable of understanding the consequences, then staff must determine if it is more helpful or harmful to allow Charlie to have dessert every night. What would you decide?

5. When would you involve family in these decisions?

6. Now, try to imagine a sexual scenario (e.g., a resident in the mild stages of dementia who wants to engage in sexual activity with another resident). Would you use substituted judgment or best interest in deciding whether to allow the activity?

Imagine the Future

Imagine yourself 50 years from now, forced by incapacity to rely on the care of others for all of your basic needs. What would you want to retain of your emotional life?

6

Inappropriate Behaviors

OBJECTIVES

- Define inappropriate behavior and the potential causes of it
- Assess inappropriate and appropriate behaviors
- Address caregiver attitudes regarding inappropriateness of sexual expression
- Provide strategies for diverting inappropriate behaviors
- Examine the issue of sexual offenders in the care home environment

*N*urse Betty was beside herself. It was the third time in a week that staff had complained to her about Clarence. Until recently, Clarence had been a model resident in the dementia wing of the nursing home where Betty was the director of nursing. All of the residents, staff, and family members loved to visit with him whenever they had the chance. He could usually be found in his wheelchair in the lobby just off the front entrance.

But something had changed. Clarence had begun unzipping his pants and masturbating, much to the consternation of anyone within sight. Because staff cared for Clarence they tried diverting his attention to something else, or they might roll him back to his room for more privacy. As time went on they were becoming fed up with his behavior, and Betty knew it was only a matter of time before she would get a complaint from family visitors.

She assembled a team of Clarence's caregivers to try to develop a plan of action. When Betty opened the floor for suggestions one staff member thought they might try putting Clarence's pants on backward, while another supported the possibility of restraints. Another said, "He doesn't do that kind of thing around me because he knows I'll slap his hand and tell him he's bad. When he acts like a child you must treat him *like a child."* Betty sadly shook her head and made a mental note to invite someone in to provide some staff education regarding resident sexuality.

WHAT ARE INAPPROPRIATE BEHAVIORS?

Until recently, long-term care staff have classified almost all forms of sexual expression by older adult residents as inappropriate. With education, staff members have begun to realize that residents have the right to express themselves sexually. Some of these activities, however, are likely to become problematic in communal living (this is true for a community of any age). Staff and ombudsmen are called upon to help solve these problems, which, if not corrected, may lead to unhappy residents, staff, and families. At their worst they may lead to legal actions against the home.

In a sense, few things can really be called inappropriate behaviors. There are just inappropriate times and places for some behaviors. One staff member calls this the "underwear in the living room" principle. In the privacy of your own home you can wear anything you want in your living room, but you probably cannot get away with it in a college dorm or in a nursing home hallway.

Definitions

Disinhibition is a lack of restraint manifested by disregard for social conventions. People who are disinhibited have a reduced capacity to control impulsive responses to situations or their environment. *Hypersexuality* is a form of disinhibition described as an abnormally high desire to engage in sexual activities. Hypersexuality refers to persistent, uninhibited sexual behavior directed at oneself or other people, and may include excessive masturbation in public and private areas, but usually involves an insatiable desire for sexual contact with others. It may also include lewd or suggestive language, fondling, flirtation, disrobing, and other overt sexual acts.

Definitions of behaviors that are seen as inappropriate are reliant on the intent of the action and are focused on intrusive behaviors (actions toward another without his or her consent), such as vulgar talk, public masturbation or nudity, and abuse. They may also include behaviors that may have more than one meaning, such as touching, hand holding, hugging, or kissing. The following is a list of inappropriate sexual behaviors that are common in residential care:

- Fondling, hugging, or kissing strangers and staff (e.g., certified nursing assistants)
- Masturbating in public
- Undressing or being naked in public
- Using sexual language
- Acting in a manner that is sexually suggestive
- Initiating or participating in sexual activity
- Aggressive or repeated sexual overtures
- Exposing oneself during personal care
- Urinating or defecating in public areas
- Requesting excessive genital care
- False accusation of sexual abuse

These behaviors more often manifest themselves in people diagnosed with some form of dementia or mental health disorder and should therefore be viewed as the result of pathological changes in the brain. Clinicians, nurses and care staff, family, and other residents may also judge some sexual expressions as inappropriate simply because of the lack of privacy in long-term care facilities.

Gender differences exist in the reporting of inappropriate behavior. Men like to touch and women like to be touched (Mayers, 1998). Women appear to want comfort and affection while men are seen as more aggressive and forceful (Nay, 1992). Staff more often cite male residents for problematic or pathological forms of sexual expression, which more than likely will trigger a consultation from a medical professional (Archibald, 1998, Ehrenfeld et al., 1999). Many more women than men live in long-term care, especially when including caregivers. This disparity creates many more opportunities for men to have cross-gender interactions, some of which could be deemed sexually inappropriate. If more men than women lived in long-term environments, would our perceptions of gender differences in sexual expression be different?

STAFF PERCEPTION OF INAPPROPRIATE BEHAVIOR

Staff at times mislabel some behaviors as inappropriate. For example, a man who wanders into a female resident's bedroom is not necessarily acting in a sexual manner. He may simply be confused or looking for someone. The stigma attached to mislabeling a resident's behavior as sexually inappropriate may linger for a long time. A resident who has been labeled as sexually aggressive may never be free of this reputation.

The prevalence of inappropriate behavior is largely dependent on whether the staff defines a sexual expression as problematic or normal. Staff mislabelings and misperceptions about sexually inappropriate behaviors can skew accounts of the frequency of such behaviors. In fact, studies have found that between 2% and 8% of residents exhibit hypersexuality, disinhibition, or sexually inappropriate actions toward others (Burns, Jacoby, & Levy, 1990; Ryden, Bossenmaier, & McLachlan, 1991; Wagner, Teri, & Orr-Rainey, 1995).

Researchers have observed the following three categories of sexual expression in long-term care (Medeiros, Rosenberg, Baker, & Onyike, 2008):

1. *Intimacy-seeking behaviors,* which are consistent with normal interpersonal behaviors that might be seen in people without dementia, but which are misplaced in social context and may be deemed inappropriate for the residential home when exhibited by people with dementia.

2. *Disinhibited behaviors,* which are rude and intrusive and would be considered inappropriate in any living situation.

3. *Nonsexual behaviors,* which are misinterpreted by staff as being of a sexual nature.

Both intimacy-seeking behaviors and disinhibition can be problematic in long-term care residences. They occur with equal frequency and may cause equal problems (Medeiros et al., 2008). Intimacy-seeking behaviors intrude on other relationships, and the couple involved in a relationship may become hostile and irritated if separated. Disinhibited behaviors, by definition, are offensive, intrusive, and inappropriate.

While the incidence of sexual expression in long-term care may be relatively low, many people, including caregivers, residents, and family members, may be impacted. Mayers (1998) found that 70% of caregivers at a state hospital had been the victim of at least one patient-initiated attempt at sexual activity in the previous year. Of the 33 caregivers interviewed, 88% had been subjected to sexually abusive language, 79% to sexual touching (breasts, buttocks, and genitals), 70% to kissing, 48% to hugging that exceeds mere affection, 30% to attempted intercourse, 18% to mouthing of breasts, and 18% to attempted oral sex.

Current research literature does not include information about the factors that influence sexual expression in people with dementia who live in residential care, which may include past sexual abuse (Sidebar 6.1). And although the frequency of sexual expressions seems to be equal between the sexes, some suggest that disinhibited behaviors occur more often in men (Ehrenfeld, Bronner, Tabak, Alpert & Bergman, 1999; Burns, Jacoby & Levy, 1990). There also seems to be a correlation

Sidebar 6.1
Adult Survivors of Sexual Abuse

One of the issues that is seldom raised in discussions of care provision for older adults is childhood or adolescent sexual abuse. Statistics of reported abuse reveal that between 12% and 40% of adults have experienced some form of abuse in their past (Walker, Torkelson, Katon, & Koss, 1993). One in five women have experienced rape, and among girls who had sex before the age of 13, 22% reported it was involuntary. Given the reluctance of older adults to share private matters or to seek care or counseling for abuse, many more cases have gone uncounted. Shame and stigma have kept many people from revealing problems related to past abuse. Because of this it was once believed that incest was so rare as to be inconsequential.

I often wonder how many of the behavior problems experienced in nursing homes may be attributed to past abuse. I have raised this issue many times when giving presentations about person-centered care and have seen staff have ah-ha moments that past abuse might explain some behaviors they have witnessed in the home.

Imagine the implications. A nurse sneaks quietly into a darkened room for a bed check. Nurse assistants, sometimes of the opposite sex, strip residents for bathing purposes. These experiences may mirror childhood nightmares. Care staff must always be sensitive to this possibility.

Previous abuse may affect resident sexuality. Persons who have been abused commonly have more physical and mental health problems than other residents. Other issues may include sleep disorders, sexual dysfunction, psychological and behavioral disorders, compulsive sexual behavior, and intolerance of or constant search for intimacy.

Staff members must be open to the possibility that a resident experienced abuse in the past and seek help from medical and mental health professionals for how to provide sensitive care. This is also a little-explored area of research that should be examined much more closely.

with increasing cognitive impairment (incidents of inappropriate sexual expression increase) (Szasz, 1983). Two small studies have tried to link types of dementia with disinhibited or intrusive sexual activity, but have been inconclusive (Nagaratnam & Gayagay, 2002; Miller, Darby, Swartz, Yener & Mena, 1995). One study of twenty residents found that all subjects who exhibited intimacy-seeking behaviors had Alzheimer's disease, and those people with a form of dementia not related to Alzheimer's disease all displayed disinhibited behaviors (Medeiros et al., 2008).

ASSESSING APPROPRIATENESS OR INAPPROPRIATENESS OF BEHAVIORS

Perhaps the first step in assessing whether a behavior is appropriate or inappropriate is to examine the biases and beliefs of the person reporting the behavior. Does the behavior raise a legitimate concern, or is the concern raised because of a personal bias about older adult sexuality or even possibly fear of litigation? Is it assumed that mildly aberrant behavior represents a lifelong eccentricity, or is dementia assumed to be the cause of the behavior?

Another important step in determining appropriateness is to examine the sexual history of the resident. This history should ideally be taken before or soon after a resident moves into a long-term care home. Some aberrant sexual behavior may be linked to a lifelong sexual pattern. If an inappropriate sexual behavior cannot be traced to a resident's sexual history, the behavior may be due to impaired judgment or impulse control stemming from a medical condition or medication. Residents who display inappropriate behaviors should have a physical examination to rule out delirium or other acute or chronic medical conditions that may be the cause.

Sexuality is a very complex brain function, and many factors can affect how people express themselves sexually. Disruptions in neural pathways related to sex drive may adversely regulate sexual activity. Many medications may blunt sex drive and in rare cases may trigger hypersexuality (Table 6.1). The temporal and frontal lobes of the brain are the centers for libido. Disinhibition and hypersexuality have been linked to dementia or brain injury in these areas of the brain (Haddad & Benhow, 1993).

Hypersexuality, on a psychological level, may simply be a cry for intimacy. Sex may be a way to compensate for cognitive and functional losses that decrease confidence and self-esteem. Being able to perform sexually, especially for men, may be a way to feel good and powerful again. What may look like sexual aggression may actually be an attempt to use physical closeness to reduce anxiety, loneliness, or fear. In other cases, staff may view residents who repeatedly want sex as being self-centered and demanding when, in fact, some people may have dementia to the extent that they quickly forget that they just had sex.

Table 6.1   Causes of Hypersexuality

Nondementia	Anticholinergic medications: thioridazine, amitriptyline, diphenhydramine; benzodiazepines; anti-Parkinson's medication; alcohol intoxication or withdrawal, acute cerebral injury, severe systemic infection; central nervous system infection; severe renal/metabolic disturbance; postictal state (the altered stage of consciousness one enters after a seizure); cardiopulmonary disease
Dementia	Alzheimer's disease; vascular dementia; dementia with Lewy bodies; frontotemporal dementia, including Pick's disease; Klüver-Bucy syndrome; Huntington's chorea; Wernicke-Korsakoff syndrome
Other	Manic phase of bipolar disorder; schizoaffective disorders; substance abuse; obsessive compulsive disorder

Source: Adapted from Lesser, Hughes, Jemelka, & Griffith (2005).

It is important to consider that a specific behavior may not arise from the same cause in different people, or even in the same person under differing circumstances. Undressing in public, for example, may be in reaction to a change in temperature, body rashes, uncomfortable clothing, or the need to go to the bathroom. Many disturbing behaviors can occur because a resident with Alzheimer's disease does not understand or misinterprets what is expected of him or her. A resident may touch him or herself in an attempt to feel intimacy or for familiarity. He or she may not be interested in sex at all and instead needs to feel the connection provided by human touch. Something about the environment may also trigger unwanted behaviors. For example, a resident with dementia sees a sign that says "wet floor," so he unzips his pants and proceeds to wet the floor.

Other sexual aggressiveness may occur when a resident misidentifies another resident as a spouse. Thinking that sexual intimacy with this person is normal, the resident with dementia is unable to understand that such attention is in fact not appropriate. The misidentified "partner" may not be willing or able to consent, which means staff will need to protect the person from potentially being victimized.

Although staff note inappropriate sexual behaviors more often in persons with dementia, this population more commonly expresses indifference and apathy regarding sexual expression.

STRATEGIES FOR ADDRESSING INAPPROPRIATE BEHAVIORS

Consider the following questions when dealing with undesirable behaviors and developing a plan of care that addresses the needs of residents (Ballard, 1995) (Activity 6.1):

- Exactly what is the resident doing?

- Does it happen frequently? Is there a pattern to this behavior?

- If so, when does it occur?

- Is the behavior sexual or does it have another cause?

- Does there appear to be a triggering incident, such as boredom or bathing?

- Have there been changes to the resident's living environment?

- Has the resident's medical condition changed and/or has a new medication been prescribed?

- Has the resident forgotten the social rules about private behaviors?

- Is the behavior an indication of a need for attention?

- Why is this behavior a problem? (safety, disruption, etc.)

- For whom is the behavior a problem—the resident, other residents, family, staff?

- Is there a risk/benefit to the behavior? Does the risk outweigh the benefit?

- Does the behavior represent a psychological need on the part of the resident (e.g., need to be reassured due to fear of abandonment, need to prove manhood)?

- Could caregivers be misinterpreting the behavior?

Remember that staff or family members frequently do not know how to handle inappropriate behaviors because of deep-seated attitudes, biases, values, and long-held beliefs about expressions of sexuality in general or more specifically in older adults. In addition, some behaviors are likely to be misidentified as being sexual in nature when in fact they are not. Whatever the answer to these questions, staff should react calmly when addressing inappropriate behaviors (Sidebar 6.2). It is important to observe the recurring behavior and devise strategies to distract, divert, or attend to the basic need that the resident may be expressing. Chart the behavior and report the progress in addressing it to the people who need to know (e.g., family, staff, attending physician).

Treatment Options

Perhaps the best treatment is prevention. It may be necessary to collect a resident's social and sexual histories upon admission, although residents are sometimes too confused or anxious and family members too embarrassed to give useful information. Openly addressing sexuality at admissions could prevent potential problems in the short term and possibly over time, and it may make addressing an issue easier later on. To assist staff in collecting the information, family members and residents should be told ahead of time that a resident's sexual history will need to be provided as part of the admissions process as well as the reasons why.

Sidebar 6.2
Pragmatic Tips

The following tips can assist staff in addressing issues regarding inappropriate sexual expression:

1. Approach the resident as an adult. Do not try to shame the person. Do not assume the resident cannot make decisions for him- or herself. Involve the resident in making decisions when appropriate. Remember that the behavior, in the case of dementia, is part of the disease. Caregivers should remind themselves not to take the behavior personally as well as not to impose a moral judgment on the situation. Ignore the behavior only if it is deemed the appropriate response to modify the behavior.

2. Modify the environment to encourage or support desired behaviors. This may require accommodations on the part of the caregivers.

3. Have staff evaluate their own beliefs or possible stereotypes about ill or aging adults expressing themselves sexually. Punitive actions to address inappropriate forms of sexual expression may arise from these beliefs rather than practical and healthy solutions. Also, getting to know a resident well can help caregivers effectively treat and prevent unwanted behaviors.

4. Chart and evaluate behaviors objectively. Residents may climb into bed with each other because they are used to sleeping with someone; the behavior may not be sexual. Consider that all behavior has meaning. Residents may be acting on feelings of discomfort, loneliness, hunger, pain, or the need to go to the bathroom.

5. Inform the family when situations or behaviors may have legal, ethical, or social consequences for the individuals involved. Include families in care planning, which should include identifying ways to meet a resident's need for affection and intimacy. Find ways to appropriately touch a resident when providing care.

Source: Adapted from Ballard (1995).

To ease the discomfort of the interview, staff could refer to it as a social history rather than a sexual history, and the questions could cover the types of relationships the resident enjoyed while living at home and the guests who could be expected to visit him or her in the long-term care home. Residents could be asked to identify the most important people in their life and what the staff could do to help them spend time with those special friends. It may be a good idea to delay this interview until a staff member has been able to develop a trusting relationship with the resident.

Behavioral Treatments

Behavioral treatments are preferable to medication. They can be staff intensive but do not have the side effects that medications may have. In addition, they help to avoid the "all-sex-is-bad" approach that many long-term care staff adopt.

Caregivers should remain calm and deliberate and should recognize the physiological or psychological origin of the behavior. Staff should not attach a stigmatizing label to a resident who exhibits inappropriate sexual behavior. Instead, staff may use stimulus control to reinforce sexual expression in the appropriate place and time. Other methods of behavioral control include having the resident wear restrictive clothing, observing the resident, and moving the resident away from the stimulus. The effectiveness of any behavioral treatment option depends on the level of staff available to work with a resident to address the behavior.

As mentioned previously, residents may use inappropriate forms of sexual expression when they feel a need for intimacy. Individualized attention and choices for appropriate expressions may help to reduce the unwanted behaviors. (Chapter 3 tells the story of a resident who regularly viewed pornography; with increased staff attention, his viewing of the material decreased.)

Observe the resident within the care environment to determine if there are cues to inappropriate behaviors. Music, television programs that are sexually suggestive, or contact with certain residents, staff, or visitors may potentially trigger inappropriate activity. For people with dementia, soothing music and "white noise" can be used to ameliorate undesirable behaviors. (See Chapter 8 for more on care environments.)

Consider the use of diversions, including activities that are personally meaningful to the resident. Some caregivers have found success with placing an apron or a pouch around a resident's waist with a few items to examine and explore.

See Sidebar 6.3 for a checklist that staff can use to assess problem sexual behaviors. Also, Activity 6.2 is an exercise in behavior mapping, an observational method of tracking environmental factors that may trigger inappropriate sexual expression.

Pharmacological Treatments

Staff should consider pharmacological treatments only after behavioral treatments have failed. Most of these treatments are hormonal. For example, medications that can decrease testosterone can effectively reduce sexual desire. Other effective hor-

Sidebar 6.3
Checklist for Treatment Options

The following checklist provides a tool for examining treatment options when a resident displays problematic sexual behaviors. The last resorts for this list are to transfer the resident to another unit or hospital for psychiatric evaluation or to use pharmacological treatments.

Checklist for Treating Problem Sexual Behaviors

☐ **Environment**

Review the staff dress code. Eliminate provocative clothing.

If undressing in the bedroom triggers a problem behavior, consider having the resident change in the bathroom.

Divert the resident's attention with conversations or activities based on his or her interests to eliminate boredom.

If resident frequently masturbates, avoid placing him or her in public areas.

If a resident masturbates in public areas, consider clothing adaptations (pants without zippers), or direct the resident to his or her room.

☐ **Psychiatric**

Treat manic or delusional behaviors and depression in residents.

Some depressed residents may reach out for comfort in ways that appear to be sexually motivated.

A resident who experiences delusions may believe another unrelated resident is a spouse.

☐ **Physical ailment (i.e., rash, infection)**

Itch from yeast infection may cause a female resident to appear as though she is masturbating.

Urinary infection or a rash may cause a resident to remove his or her clothing.

Prolapsed uterus may cause a feeling of pressure as if sitting on a ball.

Resident may be allergic to incontinence products.

☐ **Disease or disorder (Alzheimer's or dementia)**

Memory loss may cause a resident to be attracted to someone who resembles his or her spouse.

Frontal lobe dementia is associated with uninhibited sexual behaviors.

Social manners can be forgotten or become confused.

Excessive friendliness may be misinterpreted as sexual advance.

Distract night wanderers before they enter other resident bedrooms.

☐ **Unmet Needs**

Lack of self-esteem. Provide activities that lead to success. Offer praise.

Offer affection that is friendly but not sexual in nature.

Look for ways to eliminate fear by offering reassurance and familiar objects.

mones include estrogens, antiandrogens, gonadotropin-releasing analogues, and methylprogesterone acetate.

Psychotropic medications have had mixed results and include antipsychotics, beta-blockers, antianxiety agents, antimanic drugs, cholinesterase inhibitors, and benzodiazepines.

A number of ethical issues must be considered when applying a pharmacological approach to address inappropriate sexual behavior, including the resident's ability to give informed consent, the potential side effects of the medication, and the social stigma attached to the use of these drugs (some hormonal medications have been referred to as "chemical castration"). The risks and benefits should be carefully weighed and discussed with family and staff members.

In summary, the following steps can be implemented in the process of evaluating and treating inappropriate behaviors:

1. Once an incident has been reported, the interdisciplinary care team should thoroughly investigate by interviewing all relevant personnel as well as the resident and documenting findings.

2. If the findings are substantiated, call in the medical director or physician to complete a physical exam to determine whether the behavior resulted from a medical illness or condition. If found, the condition should be treated and the reported sexual behavior should be monitored.

3. If no medical condition is found, the care plan team and physician should meet with the family or guardian to discuss behavioral interventions, which would include observing and reassessing the behavior over time.

4. If behavioral interventions fail, the care plan team and physician should meet again with the family or guardian to discuss medication treatment options.

5. Administer the medication(s) and observe for side effects and behavioral response.

SEXUAL ABUSE

Staff must immediately address as a serious offense any act of sexual abuse on the part of a resident against another resident or against a staff member. Acts of sexual abuse should never be ignored or tolerated and should be carefully investigated. Staff and administrators must protect and support the safety and well-being of the abuse victim.

Sex offenders living in long-term care residences pose one risk factor in the potential sexual abuse of a resident or staff member (Sidebar 6.4). State legisla-

Sidebar 6.4
Sex Offenders in the Nursing Home

The problem of sex offenders living in long-term care homes has received little attention. In 2006, the U.S. Government Accountability Office (GAO) identified over 700 registered offenders living in long-term care. This may, however, be a conservative estimate as a watchdog group called the Perfect Cause reported as many as 1,600 registered sex offenders living in facilities with vulnerable older adults (Appleby, 2008).

Between the years of 2002 and 2006, 44 offenders living in nursing homes committed more than 50 sexual offenses (Appleby, 2008). Most laws do not require states to notify nursing homes that they have a sex offender living in their home. Further, no laws exist that require nursing homes to notify residents or their family members that a known offender lives in the home, and there is no provision in the law that says a nursing home can remove a person from the home if the home learns about the resident's classification.

Sex offenders are almost always male and less than 65 years old (GAO, 2006). They represent less than .05% of the entire long-term care population (GAO, 2006). Many of them committed crimes when they were much younger, but one researcher found that some sex offenders in long-term care had committed offenses when they were in their 80s, suggesting that it would not be safe to assume that sexual offenses are primarily committed at early ages (Bledsoe, 2004; GAO, 2006).

State legislators are attempting to pass laws to deal with this issue and to protect older residents. Some laws extend beyond resident populations to address employee screening as well. In 2005 in Michigan, researchers found that 43% of residents and 25% of long-term care staff who were charged with committing a sexual offense against a resident had prior criminal convictions (Socolof & Jordan, 2006).

Because the issue of sex offenders living in nursing homes is regulated at the state level, it is important that each nursing home review and train staff on current regulations.

tures regulate how to address the issue of sex offenders living in nursing homes. Each nursing home, therefore, must review current regulations regarding this issue.

As discussed in Chapter 5, issues of consent can come into play in dealing with the sexual abuse of a resident with dementia as well as in the case of an abuser who has dementia. It may be difficult to discern whether a resident with dementia has been sexually abused, particularly in cases of advanced dementia in which people are typically passive, nonverbal, and frequently nonambulatory. Likewise, it may be difficult to ascertain the abuser. It is important to monitor intimate relationships in the home to ensure that any sexual activity is consensual, especially if one or both of the residents has dementia.

Abuse can even occur between married couples living together in long-term care. Staff may infer that a spouse is forcing the other to have sex. More often the husband is the aggressor and the wife is submissive, a behavior that can be attributed to dementia, fear, and spousal expectations based on social conventions of the past.

Two women in an assisted living home had made numerous complaints to the administrator that Wally had been climbing into their beds. One of them stated, "When a man gets right into bed, sits down, and goes under the covers, it's sexual harassment and it has gone too far." She told management that if it happened again, she would call the police. Which is exactly what she did.

When the officer arrived he acted condescendingly and suggested that Wally had a psychological problem and that the resident should complain to the director—something she had already done several times before. The nurse and the police officer suggested that she lock her door, which she had not done because of health problems. She had wanted staff to have easy access if she needed help.

The woman felt victimized three times over, once by Wally, once by administration, and then again by the police officer. After this incident the two women who had complained about Wally were told that there were sufficient grounds to break their contracts and they were asked to leave the facility. (Frankowski and Clark [2009])

ABUSE BY NURSING HOME STAFF

One of the most disruptive and disturbing forms of inappropriate sexual expression occurs when a resident falsely accuses a staff member of sexual abuse.

Whether true or false, these allegations must be taken seriously and investigated fully. False accusations may be avoided if caregivers wear appropriate clothing, monitor their language when providing care, and frequently identify themselves to the residents who have dementia.

Of course, sometimes allegations are proven true. The threat of abuse increases in care environments where the residents are highly vulnerable (nonambulatory, nonverbal), do not have the ability to give consent, or cannot defend themselves. In addition, caregiving activities (bathing, dressing, toileting) require close physical contact with residents. Long-term care facilities should carefully screen their employees to avoid hiring sex offenders.

SUMMARY

When a resident suddenly displays an unexpected or inappropriate form of sexual expression, staff members frequently react on impulse. Their perception of the behavior may be exaggerated, and their reaction may actually be worse than the behavior that provoked it. With proper education, staff can effectively address issues of inappropriate sexual expression with greater understanding and a calmer approach. Long-term care settings can use the following systematic process to reduce or eliminate problematic forms of sexual expression:

- Gather facts.
- Search for the meaning in the behavior.
- Determine whose problem it is.
- How does the problem affect others?
- What interventions have been attempted?
- What is the desired outcome?
- What is a realistic or acceptable outcome?
- Brainstorm interventions and develop a plan of action.

REFERENCES

Appleby, J. (2008). Lawmakers look at sex offenders in nursing homes. *USA Today.* Retrieved from http://www.usatoday.com/news/nation/2008-07-24-sexoffender_N. htm.

Archibald, C. (1998). Sexuality, dementia and residential care: Managers report and response. *Health and Social Care in the Community, 6*(2), 95–101.

Ballard, E. (1995). Attitudes, myths, and realities: Helping families and professional caregivers cope with sexuality in the Alzheimer's patient. *Sexuality and Disability, 13*(3), 255–270.

Bledsoe, W. (2004). A perfect cause. Retrieved from http://www.aperfectcause. org/predator press.html

Burns, A., Jacoby, R., & Levy, R. (1990). Psychiatric phenomena in Alzheimer's disease: Disorders of behavior. *British Journal of Psychiatry, 157*(7), 86–94.

Ehrenfeld, M., Bronner, G., Tabak, N., alpert, R., & Bergmen, R. (1999). Sexuality among institutionalized elderly patients with dementia. *Nursing Ethics, 6*(2), 144–149.

Frankowski , A. C., & Clark, L. (2009). Sexuality and intimacy in assisted living: Residents' perspectives and experiences. *Sexuality Research and Social Policy, 6*(4), 25–37.

GAO (2006). Information on residents who are registered sex offenders or are paroled for other crimes. *Government Accountability Office Highlights.* Retrieved from www.gao.gov/new.items/ d06323.pdf.

Haddad, P., & Benbow, S. (1993). Sexual problems associated with dementia: Part 2. Aetiology, assessment, and treatment. *International Journal of Geriatric Psychology, 8,* 631–637.

Lesser, J., Hughes, S., Jemelka. J., & Griffith, J. (2005). Sexually inappropriate behaviors. *Geriatrics, 60*(1), 34–37.

Mayers, K. (1998). Sexuality and the demented patient. *Sexuality and Disability, 16*(3), 219–225.

Medeiros, K., Rosenberg, P., Baker, A., & Onyike, C. (2008). Improper sexual behaviors in elders with dementia living in residential care. *Dementia and Geriatric Cognitive Disorders, 26,* 370–377.

Miller, B., Darby, A., Swartz, J., Yener, G., & Mena, I. (1995). Dietary changes, compulsions and sexual behavior in frontotemporal degeneration. *Dementia, 6,* 195–199.

Nagaratnam, N., & Gayagay, G. (2002). Hypersexuality in nursing care facilities: A descriptive study. *Archives of Gerontology and Geriatrics, 35,* 195–203.

Nay, R. (1992). Sexuality and aged women in nursing homes. *Geriatric Nursing, 16*(6), 312–314.

Ryden, M., Bossenmaier, M., & McLachlan, C. (1991). Aggressive behavior in cognitively impaired nursing home residents. *Research in Nursing and Health, 14,* 87–95.

Socolof, J., & Jordan, J. (2006). Best practices for healthcare background screening. *Journal of Health Care Compliance.* Retrieved from https://www.ershire.com/ BestPracticesforHealth CareBackgroundScreening.pdf

Szasz, G. (1983). Sexual incidents in an extended care unit for aged men. *Journal of the American Geriatric Society, 31,* 407–411.

Wagner, A. W., Teri, L., & Orr-Rainey, N. (1995). Behavior problems of residents with dementia in special care units. *Alzheimer's Disease and Assorted Disorders, 9*(3), 121–127.

Walker, E., Torkelson, N., Katon, W., & Koss, M. (1993). The prevalence rate of sexual trauma in a primary care clinic. *Journal of the American Board of Family Practice, 6,* 465–471.

Case Study Discussion

At a state long-term care conference everyone was talking about the sex scandal at ABC Assisted Living. It seems that Jonas was having a problem remembering his wife. He had selected three women in the home who looked like her, and he thought he was married to each one. As if that weren't enough of a problem, he was having his wives "service" him in the hallways of the assisted living facility. When staff complained to the administrator they were told, "This is assisted living. He can do anything he wants here." Of course, the staff didn't think that was the correct response so they requested that state regulators intervene and correct the problem.

Using the list of questions to consider when dealing with undesirable behaviors, develop a plan of action that staff could have implemented to address Jonas's behavior before contacting the regulators. What would you tell this administrator about his or her response to the situation?

Behavior Mapping

Behavior mapping is an observational method for assessing the environmental factors that may trigger inappropriate sexual expression. Typically one or two staff members chart their observations over a 6-hour period. Those persons conducting the assessment should not be employees from the unit to be examined. Staff would take notes every 5 minutes about observed behaviors, activities, interactions, and mood states, as well as code each with either a positive or negative number, indicating positive or negative factors.

A simpler form of mapping would be to create a chart that lists the most problematic behaviors, along with the times of day and potential environmental influences (e.g., specific staff member providing care, time period prior to a meal, long periods of inactivity). Staff can use checkmarks to indicate when certain activities occur.

7

Lesbian, Gay, Bisexual, and Transgendered Residents

OBJECTIVES

- Define terms as applied to *lesbian, gay, bisexual,* and *transgender* (LGBT) populations
- Discuss the prevalence of LGBT individuals living in long-term care
- Describe the fear LGBTs face in long-term care
- Discuss strategies for staff sensitivity training in addressing the needs of LGBT residents

*S*am and Paul had been together for years. They had a strong "family of choice"—friends who provided them with a support network. Unexpectedly, Paul suffered a debilitating stroke. After a stay in the hospital and months of rehabilitation that did little to improve Paul's paralysis, Sam was forced to move him to a nursing home.

Sam was unsure how the staff might treat Paul had they learned he was a homosexual, so he did not reveal their true relationship. He tried not to show too much affection when staff were present. When Paul's condition worsened, the nursing staff and administration did not recognize Sam as a person who could make care decisions for Paul, and he stood by helplessly when a feeding tube was inserted, something Sam knew Paul would never have wanted.

DEFINITIONS

The following terms are used in association with the gay, lesbian, bisexual, and transgender (LGBT) population.

Homosexual. Individuals who are sexually attracted to members of their own sex. Not all those who experience sexual attraction toward members of their own sex identify themselves as being gay or homosexual.

Men who have sex with men. This phrase is frequently used to describe an identity, a community, and a behavior. With same-sex sexual behavior, however, lesbians or gays may be celibate; therefore, being gay or lesbian is a matter of identity and a much broader, more holistic concept that includes social, emotional, and political elements.

Bisexual. People who are sexually attracted to members of their own sex as well as those of the opposite sex.

Transgender. An umbrella term for people who do not conform to society's strict traditional gender categories of male and female. They may identify with a sex that does not conform to their body type, may define themselves as both female and male, or may not identify with either sex.

Transsexual. People who psychologically identify with and want to be accepted as the opposite gender. Typically this is associated with a sex-change operation.

Heterosexism. Discrimination or prejudice by heterosexuals against homosexuals. This is a system of beliefs that favors opposite-sex sexuality and relationships. Many believe that opposite-sex relationships are the norm and are, therefore, superior.

Homophobia. This is an irrational fear or hatred of or discrimination against homosexuality or homosexuals. Older gays and lesbians experience heterosexism and homophobia from the larger heterosexual community and ageism from the gay and lesbian community.

It may be difficult to find a staff member who feels comfortable leading a training program for sensitivity to the needs of the LGBT population. In this case it would be important to bring a professional to the organization to direct education. This training could be part of an inclusion program that addresses diversity in general (which is beyond the scope of this book) (Activity 7.1).

OLDER LESBIANS, GAYS, BISEXUALS, AND TRANSSEXUALS

In 1948, Dr. Alfred C. Kinsey wrote *Sexual Behavior in the Human Male* and claimed that 10% of the male population was gay. In 1993, the *Janus Report* on *Sexual Behavior* estimated that 9% of American males and 5% of females had more than "occasional" homosexual relationships. In 2000, the U.S. Census Bureau reported that homosexual couples represented less than 1% of American households while the National Gay and Lesbian Task Force estimate was 3%–8%.

Most of these estimates would put the truth at roughly 1 in every 15 or 16 adults being homosexual. Interestingly, in 2002, when Gallup polled Americans asking them to estimate the percentage of gays and lesbians in the population, the average estimates were 21% of men and 22% of women, or 1 in every 5 adults (Robinson, 2002). Only about 40% of transgender people and just 16% of bisexual people are completely or mostly out (have identified themselves publicly as being such), compared to 74% of gay men and 76% of lesbians (MetLife, 2010).

According to a 2010 AARP survey of 1,200 LGBT persons between the ages of 45 and 64, half of the respondents said their family members were "completely" or "very" accepting of their lives as LGBT people. These percentages, however, varied significantly between those who were lesbian, gay, bisexual, and transgendered. The majority of lesbians and gay men said their families were accepting, but this was less true for bisexuals (24%) and transgendereds (42%). When asked about how careful they had to be to hide their sexual orientation, bisexuals were much more likely to say they were guarded with nearly everyone with whom they came in contact.

LGBTs experience the same losses as other older people—loss of career, family and friends, and good health. Like most American older adults they also experience ageism. LGBTs may have other concerns as well. They are more than two-and-a-half times more likely to live alone, twice as likely to be single, and four-and-a-half times more likely to have no children to call upon when in need. Despite the fact that most live alone, they do not consider themselves lonely or isolated.

Their social networks consist of "families of friends" or "families of choice" that serve as buffers during times of need. Older gays overwhelmingly consider friends rather than family as the providers of social support, which is different from older heterosexuals. This may be because of the rejection of family or because of trying to hide their sexual orientation from relatives or because of childlessness.

Older LGBTs' desire for companionship and involvement in sexual relationships is similar to that of heterosexual people. Some researchers have found gender differences in how lesbians and gays view homosexuality (Golden, 1996; Sears, 1989). A lesbian is more likely to describe a homosexual as being a "person who shares intimate love with a person of the same sex," while a gay man is more likely to define a homosexual as a "person who has sex with a person of the same sex" (Sears, 1989, p. 425). Just as has been observed among heterosexuals, women are more likely to romanticize relationships, whereas men sexualize them.

Most of the research literature has focused on older gay men. Stereotypes of older gays include feeling lonely and isolated, being oversexed, experiencing mental health problems, and feeling excluded from the gay youth culture. There has been little evidence to support these stereotypes. In fact, older gays are no more prone to depression or sadness than heterosexual men. The oversexed stereotype is likely the result of people thinking of homosexuality primarily in terms of sexual activity and not as a cultural, emotional, and psychological concept.

Because of the gay community's emphasis on youth, older gays are considered elderly by other homosexuals at an earlier age than heterosexual adults. Older homosexuals are less likely to socialize outside the gay community than are younger gay men. A 1980 study found that one in four older gay men surveyed were in long-term relationships, which is significant because they are more likely to be caregivers given their lack of ties to other potential caregivers (i.e., family members or children) and because of fear of discrimination in formal health care settings (Bennett & Thompson, 1980).

In addition to being homosexual, some may also be members of a minority, meaning they may face racism as well as ageism and homophobia. Because of the risks of potentially facing multiple forms of discrimination, many LGBTs have chosen to be silent about their sexual orientation or gender identity. The act of concealing one's sexual identify over time can become unhealthy, as it reinforces the notion to others that what someone is doing or experiencing is wrong and as it becomes increasingly difficult for the person to hide from others an important part of who he or she is.

For those who have been open about their sexuality, there is the belief that having to cope with a painful coming out may make older LGBTs stronger and more able to cope with aging. When the 2010 AARP survey asked about this ability to cope, respondents noted two categories: personal and interpersonal strengths and overcoming adversity. Personal and interpersonal strengths included the following:

- More accepting of others
- Not taking anything for granted

- Being more resilient or having a stronger inner strength
- Being more self-reliant
- Being more careful in legal and financial matters
- Having a family of choice

Overcoming adversity included the following traits:

- Knowing how cruel society can be
- Being able to cope with discrimination

More than a quarter of the respondents said that their sexual orientation and/or gender identity did not help them prepare for aging.

Older adults' ability to be open about their sexual orientation and gender identity is closely related to their historical past. Those living in nursing homes today came of age during World War II. The war brought many lesbians together for the first time. Gay and lesbian bars opened in urban areas, but they were repeatedly raided and the patrons were arrested. Homosexuality was identified as a mental disorder, and some gays and lesbians were subjected to shock treatments in attempts by family members to cure them.

It has become much more socially acceptable for same-sex couples to cohabitate. Younger gays and lesbians today can openly enter into civil unions in a handful of states, become parents, and enjoy many civil rights. Between 1992 and 2002, the acceptance of gays and lesbians improved (Robinson, 2002). In 2010, a Gallup poll estimated 52% acceptance of gay and lesbian relations based on a random sample of 1,029 Americans over the age of 18, compared to 38% in 1992.

Media portrayals of gays and lesbians have increased and emphasized positive models. Many famous people have come out and spoken about their life experiences. In recent times there has been a drive for celebrities to come out to help younger people who suffer ridicule and abuse and who may choose to take their own life because of it. These social movements would suggest that LGBTs will be much more open about their sexuality by the time they move to a long-term care setting.

LGBTs IN LONG-TERM CARE

In American culture people are presumed to be heterosexual until proven otherwise. Even though social gerontology increasingly recognizes aging issues for LGBTs, older LGBTs may still be invisible, and planning and service provisions in long-term care do not address their needs. This has been called the "heteronormativity" of long-term care services.

If we estimate that 1 in 15 older adults is gay or lesbian, then in the average nursing home with 50 residents we could expect at least three residents to be gay or lesbian. Estimates of the homosexual population are difficult because neither the U.S. Census Bureau nor other population studies ask about sexual orientation. One study estimates that roughly 120,000 to 300,000 older gays and lesbians will reside in nursing homes by 2030 (this does not consider other institutions) (Cohen, Curry, Jenkins, Walker, & Hogstel, 2008).

Only about 14% of older LGBTs are open about their sexuality (Heaphy, Yip, & Thompson, 2003). This may be partially due to the fact that roughly only 35% believe that health professionals harbor positive attitudes toward LGBT people, and only 16% trust health professionals to be knowledgeable about their lifestyle (Heaphy Yip, & Thompson, 2003). While many older adults have struggled and fought to come out about their sexuality, many believe that they must return to the closet to protect themselves in long-term care settings.

Older LGBTs may remember a time when they were labeled "sick by doctors, immoral by clergy, unfit for the military, and a menace by the police" (Kochman, 1997, p. 8). Homosexual activity has been criminalized in the past. Life-course perspectives link childhood and early adolescent events to later experiences in adulthood. Older LGBTs have faced a lifetime of abuse and rejection at worst and marginalization at best. Because of their past, unless they see evidence of affirmation, they will expect the worst.

In a 2006 survey of the LGBT community, 19% of the respondents had little to no confidence that they would be treated well in old age by medical personnel, and more than a third had declined to disclose their sexual orientation to their health care provider (MetLife Mature Market Institute, 2006).

There are a number of reasons for the concerns of older LGBTs. First, as younger adults they experienced structural and institutional homophobia, heterosexism, and antigay violence with respect to health care, housing, employment, and civil rights. As older adults they have also experienced disparities in coverage of same-sex couples under policies regulating Social Security, Medicare, and private pension plans. Those in the LGBT population do not qualify for survivor benefits through Social Security or Medicaid spousal impoverishment protection. Because of these restrictions older LGBTs are reluctant to access formal caregiving networks when their family or friends can no longer care for them.

Older LGBTs are also more likely to avoid routine health care due to their lack of confidence in how professional care providers view them. Aging-related conditions such as hearing loss and cardiovascular disease typically are diagnosed much later among gay seniors, a factor that complicates their care.

The "medico–moral alliance" that has been used to criminalize, pathologize, and present homosexuality as morally deviant has been the stated reason LGBTs return to the closet in institutional care. Seventy-three percent of gay and lesbian survey respondents stated that discrimination occurred in retirement communities, and over a third said they would go back into the closet if they were forced to move into one (Johnson, Jackson, Arnette, & Koffman, 2005). As a result, older LGBTs delay moving into long-term care, which forces family members or family members of choice to address more of their care needs to compensate.

Stein, Beckerman, and Sherman (2010) found that the fears and concerns of the LGBT population about entering into long-term care fall into four themes: fear of caregiver neglect or rejection; fear of not being accepted by other residents; concern about offending staff or other residents (by revealing sexual orientation); and a preference for gay-friendly residential options in long-term care.

Those potentially facing long-term care fear that if nursing home staff are informed of their sexual orientation, they will not receive equal or adequate care. These older LGBTs believe that most staff come from a culture that does not accept their sexual orientation. Examples of homophobic prejudice include staff who refuse to bathe LGBT residents; staff who threaten to reveal or who choose to reveal a resident's sexual orientation to other staff members and residents; gay or lesbian couples who are separated without regard to their long-term relationship; and medical treatments given without consulting a gay or lesbian partner. A 1995 article in *Contemporary Long Term Care* shared the story of two older male residents who were discovered engaging in oral sex (Parsons, 1995). The two were separated and within a day one of the two men was transferred to a psychiatric ward and placed in restraints.

These biases are well documented as widespread in the health care setting. A 1994 survey conducted by the Gay and Lesbian Medical Association found that two-thirds of doctors and medical students were aware of bias and prejudice in caregiving for LGBTs (Schatz & O'Hanlan, 1994). Nearly 90% reported hearing disparaging remarks made about LGBT patients.

Interestingly, the more recent 2010 AARP study found that LGBTs from the baby boomer cohort expressed far less fear of being treated poorly in long-term care. Of the 1,200 people surveyed only 10% feared discrimination because of their sexual orientation and/or gender identity. The study authors speculated that this reduced fear is because the baby boomer cohort has become accustomed to demanding respect.

LGBT fears of not being accepted or being rejected extend to other residents, especially a roommate who may dislike "different" people. Older adults, because of their lack of education regarding sexuality in general and homosexuality specifically, may have more homophobic tendencies.

LGBTs also worry about offending other people, so they feel they need to hide their sexual orientation (forcing themselves back into the closet). Those who have had lifelong relationships and may be grieving the loss of a loved one may not get the psychological interventions they need because they feel they cannot talk about these relationships. Returning to the closet is troubling for those who have lived open lives because they are concealing a critical part of their identity in order to feel physically and emotionally safe in the long-term care setting. Concealing their sexual identity also limits lesbians' and gays' ability to integrate their life experiences across their life spans and to take meaning from their lives, which may lead to greater levels of depression and physical health problems. If LGBTs retreat back into the closet, health care professionals cannot understand and address the challenges these residents face.

While some LGBTs may express a preference for gay-friendly residential options for long-term care, they have several reasons for not choosing to move to communities of this type. Many may lack the financial resources; typically these communities do not accept Medicaid reimbursement and can be very expensive. These communities may also be long distances from friends or family. Further, many LGBTs express the desire not to live in a segregated community.

It should be noted that the barriers to sexuality and sexual expression that older LGBTs face in long-term care are in addition to those they face based on the ageist beliefs of others, specifically staff (see Chapter 2). Partner availability is a primary barrier for older adults in general, but it may be even more so for LGBT residents because long-term care staff often ignore and stigmatize the sexual needs of this group even more than they do the needs of non-LGBT residents. Moving to long-term care housing, therefore, may be more traumatizing for the LGBT elder than it is for the heterosexual older adult (Sidebar 7.1; Activity 7.2).

BISEXUAL AGING

Probably the least amount of research regarding sexual orientation and gender identity has been conducted with people who identify themselves as bisexual. Much of the disparity has been due to the fact that bisexuals perceive themselves as being the least accepted and, therefore, have not been open about their sexuality. It has also been assumed that the bisexual experience is similar to that of either the homosexual or heterosexual experience.

The 2010 AARP study found this to be a misconception. According to the report, bisexuals have the lowest rates of being out and finding acceptance, have significantly fewer friends, are twice as guarded with other people about their sexuality, and are far less likely to say that being LGBT was an important part of their identity.

Sidebar 7.1
Kansas State University Center on Aging Research

Research at the Center on Aging at Kansas State University revealed that only three nursing homes of the 85 that responded asked questions regarding sexual orientation as part of the admissions process (Doll, Bolender, & Hoffman, 2011). The written responses to this question were enlightening. One administrator mentioned that forms had been modified to include partner relationships. Another home used the same policy as the military's "don't ask, don't tell." Several said that they left the door open for residents or their family members to volunteer this information, but they did not ask for it (some felt it was none of their business). Two of the responses demonstrated bias or naïveté on the part of the survey participant. One said, "This is a rural area, most are hetrosexual [*sic*]." Another stated that staff were aware of problem behaviors on the part of some residents, such as talking inappropriately or masturbating, but that they were not aware that there were any gays and lesbian residents in the home. This statement seemed to indicate that staff would view LGBT residents as a problem (e.g., "We've got some kinds of problems, but we don't have that one.").

Twenty-two percent of respondents were aware of an LGBT resident within the facility. When asked how they found out, nearly all respondents said that the resident had divulged the information. One comment surprised us: "They lived together prior to admission and families wanted them separate. We let the residents choose to live together because they were both cognitive."

TRANSGENDER AGING

Because of the stigma attached to being transgendered, there is very little information about the number of people who fall into this category. The majority of transgendered individuals do not self-identify because of fear of ostracism. As a consequence, little research has been conducted on this population. Even when studies are labeled "LGBT," little is offered about those who are transgendered.

Roughly 25,000 U.S. citizens have undergone sexual reassignment surgery (SRS). The American Psychiatric Association's *Diagnostic and Statistical Manual of Mental Disorders* has placed the prevalence of SRS at 1 in 30,000 male-to-female transsexuals and 1 in 100,000 female-to-male transsexuals, meaning that there could be 175,000 to 200,000 transgendered people in America today.

Transgendered individuals are at risk for experiencing some form of discrimination and abuse in their lifetime. The *National Transgender Discrimination Survey Report on Health and Health Care* reported that 28% of the transgendered individuals surveyed had experienced some form of harassment or violence within a medical setting (Grant et al., 2010).

While little research exists about these individuals, we do know that they experience some unique challenges relative to health care that fall into the following three categories:

1. *Barriers to health care.* Many fear bias and denial of care by health care professionals and choose to delay or even refuse to seek help as a result. A higher percentage of transgendered individuals are uninsured compared with the general population.

2. *Health issues associated with the transgender experience.* Transgendered individuals are much more likely to be the victims of abuse and violence. They also experience higher rates of HIV and risky sexual behavior. One report found that no safe-sex educational materials have been developed for this population (Healthy People, 2010). Transgendered individuals use and abuse substances at a much higher rate than the general population. They also report thinking about suicide more frequently and experience higher rates of depression.

3. *Health problems specific to the transgender population.* Other health issues of concern for transgendered elders include blood clots, stroke, polycystic ovarian syndrome, osteoporosis, high cholesterol, liver disease, and diabetes. Many of these conditions are associated with the use of hormonal treatments. Fearing the rejection of the medical profession, some transgendered individuals will obtain hormones from friends, street corners, or Internet sites. These individuals are not monitored for the effects of these hormones, sometimes with fatal results. Some may use injected silicone, again without medical supervision and with associated risk results.

STAFF SENSITIVITY TO LGBTs IN LONG-TERM CARE

"This is Kansas. We don't have any sexual orientation here." This comment was made by a respondent to a Kansas State University Center on Aging survey of nursing home administrators and social service staff as to whether admissions forms ask about sexual orientation (Doll, Bolender, & Hoffman, 2011). The rise of privacy concerns has made service providers feel that sexuality is none of their business. This feeling may also arise from the fact that sexuality is often seen as sexual behavior rather than relating to a person's broader personal, social, and cultural identity. Caregivers must see resident sexuality as more than biology or behavioral activity to be able to respect it. Just as education and awareness can overcome ageist beliefs, the same principles can be used to help staff learn to be more sensitive to the needs of LGBT residents. Obviously the survey respondent who made the aforementioned comment might have benefited from some basic information about the prevalence of LGBTs in the American population—and, more specifically, in Kansas.

Caregivers tend to assume that residents are heterosexual and may make insensitive comments based on these assumptions. Alternative language should be introduced (e.g., partner instead of husband or wife). Training should be offered that teaches culturally competent and affirmative practices. LGBTs want gay-friendly staff, characterized as not assuming heterosexuality, treating all residents with dignity and respect, and honoring residents for the lives they have lived.

Staff should be trained to acknowledge LGBTs through respect and acceptance. They need to be taught to support intimate relationships (Activity 7.3). LGBTs do not seem to want to live in segregated communities; they do, however, like the option of having a wing or floor that is LGBT friendly because it feels safer. Partners should have the option to share a room. It might also be important to provide bereavement groups and support groups specific to the LGBT population.

DEVELOPING LGBT-FRIENDLY COMMUNITIES

How can a long-term care home become more accepting of the LGBT community? A good place to start is with an assessment (Activity 7.4). The home should prominently display antidiscrimination policies that specify sexual orientation and gender identity. The statement "We do not discriminate on grounds of sexual orientation or gender identity" sets a positive tone for residents, staff, and visitors. Staff should review the home's literature, including brochures, pamphlets, and website, for evidence of inclusion, such as pictures of people with diverse sexual orientation. Do pictures hanging in common areas only depict heterosexual couples? Does the home supply reading material that may be appropriate for the LGBT population? Do staff members use the term *partner* instead of *husband* or *wife*?

Intake and assessment forms should be examined for gender-exclusive language. They can be modified to be gender neutral, such as including *domestic part-*

ner or *same-sex partner* to reflect a broader interpretation of family. The forms should clearly state that the information is confidential and that the resident's privacy will be respected. Staff should recognize the same-sex partner's or domestic partner's legal legitimacy as the person to notify as the next of kin, if such designations have been addressed by state policies. Resident rights must be observed, including those of same-sex partners in decision making and care planning.

LGBTs should not be forced to "come out" at admission. On the other hand, having to go back into the closet can be damaging to an individual's personal identity and emotional and psychological well-being. Residents and their visiting partners or friends should know that it is safe to be open about their identity and their relationships. The loss of support networks may make the adjustment to the new, potentially hostile environment even more difficult.

Staff training, brochures, and other materials pertaining to LGBT residents should be specific to each group. Transgendered persons have very different circumstances relative to health care, and it is not appropriate to use materials or programs that were designed for another population. For example, training materials for HIV prevention may not exist for the transgendered adult and may have to be created in-house. Policies should be developed that include consequences for discrimination. Regular staff training should be conducted, and LGBT staff should be recruited. Leaders of the organization must be committed to inclusion. Activities programming within the long-term care environment should also be inclusive.

DISCUSSION

Return to the story at the beginning of the chapter. What could be done to make Paul and Sam feel more comfortable with their situation? What policies might be needed to ensure that Paul's and Sam's needs are met as equitably as those of other residents? Do staff at your home have a heteronormative approach to care planning and service provisions—do they assume that all residents are heterosexual?

SUMMARY

The losses associated with moving into a long-term care setting are compounded for the LGBT population. Older LGBTs have faced a lifetime of discrimination, many live alone without family support, and most have a distrust of the medical community. These individuals are fearful of the treatment they may receive in an institutional environment. After struggling to come out and live openly, many LGBTs may choose to return to the closet to avoid discriminatory actions.

These fears cannot be alleviated without developing specific policies and educating and training staff to address the needs of the LGBT population. Long-term care organizations should thoroughly assess their environment; admissions forms; pamphlets, posters, and brochures; resident rights policies; and staff training procedures to become more inclusive and honor the needs of the LGBT population.

REFERENCES

AARP (2010). Still out, still aging: The MetLIfe study of lesbian, gay, bisexual and transgender baby boomers. Westport, CT: MetLife.

Bennett, K., & Thompson, N. (1980). Social and psychological functioning of the aging male homosexual. *British Journal of Psychiatry, 137*, 361–370.

Cohen, H., Curry, L. C., Jenkins, D., Walker, C., & Hogstel, M. (2008). Older lesbians and gay men: Long-term care issues. *Annals of Long-Term Care,* 33–38. Retrieved from http://www.annalsoflongtermcare.com/article/8315.

Doll, G., Bolender, B., & Hoffman, H. (2011). Sexuality in nursing homes: Practice and policy. Manuscript submitted for publication.

Gallup. (2010). Americans' acceptance of gay relations crosses the 50% threshold. Retrieved from www.gallup.com/poll/135764/americans-acceptance-gay-relations-crosses-threshold. aspx.

Golden, C. (1996). What's in a name? Sexual self-identification among women. In *The Lives of Lesbians, Gays, and Bisexuals: Children to Adults,* Ritch C. Savin-Williams and Kenneth M. Cohen (Eds.), pp. 229–249. Fort Worth, TX: Harcourt Brace College.

Grant, J. M., Mottet, L. A., Tanis, J., Herman, J. L., Harrison, J., & Keisling, M. (2010). *National transgender discrimination survey report on health and health care,* Retrieved from http://www.scribd.com/doc/46207496/National-Transgender-Discrimination-Survey-Report-on-Health-and-Health-Care.

Healthy People. (2010). The LGBT health issues companion document. Retrieved from http://www.nalgap.org/PDF/Resources/HP2010CDLGBTHealth.pdf.

Heaphy, B., Yip, A., & Thompson, D. (2003). *Lesbian, gay and bisexual lives over 50.* Nottingham: York House Publications.

Janus, S. S., & Janus, C. L. (1993). *The Janus report.* New York: John Wiley.

Johnson, M. J., Jackson, N. C., Arnette, J. K., & Koffman, S. D. (2005). Gay and lesbian perceptions of discrimination in retirement care facilities. *Journal of Homosexuality, 49*(2), 83–102.

Kinsey, A. C. (1948). *Sexual behavior in the human male.* Bloomington: Indiana University Press.

Kochman, A. (1997). Gay and lesbian elderly: Historical overview and implications for social work practice. *Journal of Gay and Lesbian Social Services, 6*(1), 1–10.

MetLife Mature Market Institute (2006). *Out and aging: The MetLife study of lesbian and gay baby boomers.* Westport, CT: Author.

MetLife. (2010). Still out, still aging: The MetLife study of lesbian, gay, bisexual, and transgender baby boomers. Retrieved from www.metlife.com/assets/cao/ mmi/publications/ studies/ 2010/mmi-still-out-still-aging.pdf.

Parsons, Y. (1995). Private acts, public places. *Contemporary Long Term Care, 18*(3), 48–49, 51, 53–55.

Robinson, J. (2002). What percentage of the population is gay? Retrieved from http://www.gallup.com/poll/6961/what-percentage-population-gay.aspx.

Schatz, B., & O'Hanlan, K. (1994). Anti-gay discrimination in medicine: Results of a national survey of lesbian, gay and bisexual physicians. San Francisco: American Association of Physicians for Human Rights.

Sears, J. (1989). The impact of gender and race on growing up lesbian and gay in the south. *NWSA Journal, 1,* 422–457.

Stein, G. L., Beckerman, N. L., & Sherman, P. A. (2010). Lesbian and gay elders and long-term care: Identifying the unique psychosocial perspectives and challenges. *Journal of Gerontological Social Work, 53*(5), 421–435.

U. S. Census Bureau (2000). Profiles of general demographic characteristics. Retrieved from http://www2.census.gov/census_2000/datasets/demographic_ profile/0_United_States/2kh00.pdf.

Wilkerson, G. (n.d.). What we don't know: The unaddressed health concerns of the transgendered. Trans-Health.com. Retrieved from www.trans-health.com/displayarticle.php?aid=7.

Connect the Dots

The goal of this activity is to demonstrate how difficult it can be to see things that are outside our own perspective.

Hand out copies of the dots worksheet found on the next page. Ask participants to follow the instructions on the worksheet. Allow about 5 minutes to complete the puzzle. Provide the solution (on the last page of the activity). Lead a discussion using these questions:

- Few people choose to think outside the box with this activity. Why is this difficult?

- To answer this puzzle correctly you had to draw outside the lines. This is similar to the way that we have to reach outside our own beliefs when we interact with persons who are different from ourselves.

- How can you apply this exercise to how you might feel about lesbians, gays, bisexuals, and transgendered individuals?

- How do you think it makes LGBTs feel when staff make assumptions that everyone is heterosexual?

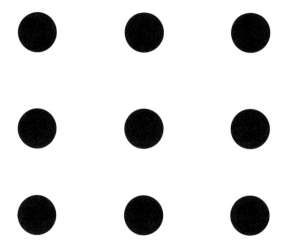

The goal of the "nine dots" puzzle is to link all nine dots using four straight lines or less, without lifting the pen and without tracing the same line more than once. The solution is on the next page.

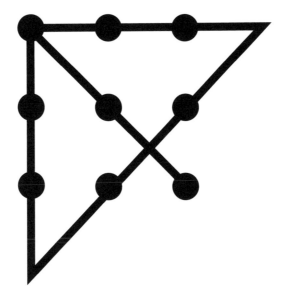

Activity 7.2

Gen Silent

View the short version of the film *Gen Silent,* available online (see For Further Information at the back of the book). This video shows interviews with older homosexuals who express their fears of moving to a nursing home facility.

Take some time to reflect on what you have seen. Imagine yourself as one of the people featured. What could you have done to advocate for yourself? What historical events or activities led to the fear of being ill treated in a home? What can you personally do to improve this situation for future residents?

Sexuality and Long-Term Care: Understanding and Supporting the Needs of Older Adults, by Gayle Appel Doll (Copyright 2012, by Health Professions Press, Inc.)

What Is Your Comfort Zone?

Directions: This a self-assessment exercise. While some of the situations on the questionnaire may or may not have been your experience, try as best you can to put yourself in the situation and determine your comfort level. Circle the answer (Strongly Agree, Agree, Disagree, or Strongly Disagree) that best describes your feelings. This exercise can be used to better know and understand what your attitudes and beliefs are in caring for or working with lesbian, gay, bisexual, or transgender (LGBT) individuals.

1. I would feel comfortable working closely with a lesbian, gay, bisexual, or transgender colleague or fellow employee.
    Strongly Agree   Agree   Disagree   Strongly Disagree

2. I am comfortable around homosexuals unless they flaunt their lifestyle.
    Strongly Agree   Agree   Disagree   Strongly Disagree

3. I would feel comfortable if I found myself attracted to members of my own gender as well as members of the other gender.
    Strongly Agree   Agree   Disagree   Strongly Disagree

4. I would feel uncomfortable knowing that one of my fellow employees is transgendered.
    Strongly Agree   Agree   Disagree   Strongly Disagree

5. If I saw two men holding hands in public, I would feel disgusted.

   Strongly Agree   Agree   Disagree   Strongly Disagree

6. I would feel flattered knowing that someone of my own gender was attracted to me.

   Strongly Agree   Agree   Disagree   Strongly Disagree

7. I would feel uncomfortable if I found out that my adult son feels he is actually a woman.

   Strongly Agree   Agree   Disagree   Strongly Disagree

8. Lesbian/gay teachers should not be "out" at school.

   Strongly Agree   Agree   Disagree   Strongly Disagree

9. I would feel comfortable if I learned that my child is lesbian, gay, or bisexual.

   Strongly Agree   Agree   Disagree   Strongly Disagree

10. It would disturb me to find out that my doctor is a lesbian.

   Strongly Agree   Agree   Disagree   Strongly Disagree

11. I would feel comfortable if my best friend of the same gender told me he/she is gay/lesbian.

   Strongly Agree   Agree   Disagree   Strongly Disagree

12. I would feel uncomfortable knowing that my son's male teacher is gay.

   Strongly Agree   Agree   Disagree   Strongly Disagree

13. I would feel uncomfortable knowing that my neighbor is a transsexual.

   Strongly Agree   Agree   Disagree   Strongly Disagree

14. I would feel comfortable being seen at the Pride parade.

   Strongly Agree   Agree   Disagree   Strongly Disagree

15. I would be disturbed if I found out that my best friend's husband likes dressing in women's clothing.

   Strongly Agree   Agree   Disagree   Strongly Disagree

Sexuality and Long-Term Care: Understanding and Supporting the Needs of Older Adults, by Gayle Appel Doll
(Copyright 2012, by Health Professions Press, Inc.)

16. I would feel comfortable working with residents who identify as LGBT.

    Strongly Agree   Agree   Disagree   Strongly Disagree

17. I feel knowledgeable about LGBT issues as related to my area of service.

    Strongly Agree   Agree   Disagree   Strongly Disagree

18. I'm willing to accept that I don't know everything about LGBT issues but am committed to finding out.

    Strongly Agree   Agree   Disagree   Strongly Disagree

Source: Adapted from Breaking Barriers Through Education, Rainbow Resource Centre, Winnipeg, Rainbow Health Educational Toolkit Workshop #2 Handouts.

Organization Inclusion Assessment for LGBT Population

This assessment may be completed by several persons from the organization. The results should be compared and, if discrepancies occur, should be explored. "No" and "Don't know" responses constitute areas for improvement.

ENVIRONMENT

1. Does your long-term care organization display an antidiscrimination policy with a positive statement of equal care such as, "We do not discriminate regardless of sexual orientation or gender identity?"

   YES   NO   DON'T KNOW

2. Does your home display pamphlets, posters, and brochures that include positive images of people of diverse sexual orientation and gender identities rather than strictly depicting heterosexual relationships?

   YES   NO   DON'T KNOW

3. Do caregivers use inclusive language, for example, using the term *partner* instead of *husband* and *wife*?

   YES   NO   DON'T KNOW

Sexuality and Long-Term Care: Understanding and Supporting the Needs of Older Adults, by Gayle Appel Doll (Copyright 2012, by Health Professions Press, Inc.)

ADMISSION

1. Does the admissions form include gender-neutral options such as *domestic partner* or *same-sex partner* along with options to choose male/female/both/neither?
   YES   NO   DON'T KNOW

2. Does your home adopt each resident's definition of "family," which may include, but not be limited to, significant others, relatives by blood, same-sex partners, or spouses?
   YES   NO   DON'T KNOW

3. Is it obvious to the resident that confidentiality is protected and privacy is respected?
   YES   NO   DON'T KNOW

RESIDENT RIGHTS

1. Do staff members use gender-neutral questions to ask about relationships and sexual behaviors?
   YES   NO   DON'T KNOW

2. If a resident's same-sex partner visits the resident, is the partner acknowledged or included in the same way a heterosexual partner is?
   YES   NO   DON'T KNOW

3. When a transgender person enters the home do you address them as their chosen gender?
   YES   NO   DON'T KNOW

4. Do caregivers treat information regarding sexual orientation or gender identity as highly sensitive information?
   YES   NO   DON'T KNOW

POLICIES

1. Does your organization have a written antidiscrimination policy with specific reference to sexual orientation and gender identity that includes written sign-off on policies by all employees?
   YES   NO   DON'T KNOW

2. Does your organization have policies, which include consequences, to deal with employee or client complaints of discrimination or harassment, and is there a follow-up process?
   YES   NO   DON'T KNOW

3. Does your organization have mechanisms to ensure that nondiscrimination policies are appropriately conveyed to all residents, including those with disabilities or those for whom English is not their primary language?
   YES   NO   DON'T KNOW

4. Do you have written confidentiality policies that explicitly include sexual orientation and gender identity?
   YES   NO   DON'T KNOW

5. Does your organization have policies in place pertaining to the training of all staff and new employees regarding the health issues faced by the LGBT community?
   YES   NO   DON'T KNOW

STAFF

1. Have all staff had awareness training about LGBT issues?
   YES   NO   DON'T KNOW

2. Have all staff and all new hires had training to identify and address health issues that may particularly affect members of the LGBT community, and is this training ongoing?
   YES   NO   DON'T KNOW

Sexuality and Long-Term Care: Understanding and Supporting the Needs of Older Adults, by Gayle Appel Doll (Copyright 2012, by Health Professions Press, Inc.)

3. Are members of the LGBT community actively recruited as potential staff members?

YES   NO   DON'T KNOW

4. Are employees who identify themselves as LGBT entitled to the same terms and conditions of employment as all others (e.g., employee benefits)?

YES   NO   DON'T KNOW

Identify areas of concern, such as creating an inclusive environment, admission procedures, or resident and staff rights and policies. Determine actions that the organization will take to improve areas of concern in the next 6 weeks, the next 6 months, and the next year. Yes responses identify strengths, whereas No and Don't Know responses indicate areas needing attention.

Source: Adapted from the Canadian Rainbow Health Coalition.

Environment

OBJECTIVES

- Discuss resident privacy rights related to the care envirnonment
- Highlight care environments that compromise or support intimate relationships
- Identify regulations that define care environments in relation to resident privacy
- Discuss private versus public rooms
- Discuss resident privacy related to visits
- Present policy options to support resident privacy through the care environment

on and Carol were visiting his mother, Shirley, in the nursing home one Sunday afternoon. Shirley shared a room with Mona. On this particular day Mona's husband had also come to visit. The curtain between the two beds was drawn, and it wasn't long before Don and Carol heard the unmistakable sounds of lovemaking. Don was horrified when the husband's foot thrust through the curtain beside him. When questioned, Shirley affirmed that this was not the first time this had occurred. Don went to lodge a complaint with the head nurse, Paul. The next day, Paul called together a team of caregivers to consider how best to handle the situation.

PRIVACY IN LONG-TERM CARE

Bauer (1999) conceptualized privacy as designated space and time that people can call their own and that does not have to be shared with other people except by

---

The sections on pages 185–198 were contributed by Migette L. Kaup, M. Arch., Associate Professor, Interior Design Program in the Department of Apparel, Textiles, and Interior Design, Kansas State University.

choice. Control over privacy is important to people living in long-term care because, for the most part, they often do not have it. Residents are seen as "old and
powerless," and after a short period living in an institutional environment they
come to believe that they are not worthy or capable of having any power or control over the simplest of activities in their lives. Unlocked door policies, evening
bed checks by staff, roommates, and staff access to all medical and health-related
information are all hindrances to a resident's privacy. While research shows that
residents are more satisfied with private rooms (Calkins & Cassella, 2007), having
one does not always ensure that privacy will be honored.

The environmental considerations discussed in this chapter focus more on
nursing homes. Assisted living environments are designed to afford residents the
privacy and autonomy they desire. Private rooms allow residents a degree of privacy and the ability to have intimate relationships. Caregiver respect for privacy
varies, however, in long-term care settings. Residents are dependent on caregivers
to provide and maintain their privacy, but not all caregivers respectfully comply.

This chapter covers environmental design considerations that may enhance
privacy for intimate relationships and sexual expression. It also covers staff practices that inhibit privacy and includes suggestions to address privacy concerns, including a visitation room for conjugal visits.

History of Nursing Home Design

Prior to the passage of Medicare in 1965, people with chronic illnesses were cared
for and lived in hospitals until they died, sometimes staying there for years. "Old
folks" homes at that time were custodial and not equipped to provide medical
care. Government funding of long-term care limited the time a patient could stay
and be covered financially, which meant that some people would eventually need
a place to go. Post World War II, the growth of an aging population and the need
for higher quality health care created a need for a new long-term care housing situation. After the passage of Medicare, long-term health care increasingly came to
be seen as the proverbial pot of gold and thousands of nursing homes were developed. The government offered subsidized loans and handed out blueprints. All
nursing homes looked alike. With little government regulation and oversight,
nursing home construction quality and design standards were poor. They were
modeled after hospitals, and like hospitals the emphasis was placed on the treatment of residents' disease conditions.

The primary design focus of these homes was to keep residents safe and to facilitate their care. As a result, residents were afforded only limited privacy. Homes
were either X or V or wheel shaped, with all corridors or hallways leading from a

central nurses' station. All rooms could be viewed from this center so that the residents could be observed at all times. An additional limit on privacy was that all rooms were shared (as they are in hospitals) to cut down on construction costs.

Clearly, nursing home design was initially intended to facilitate medical treatments and basic care. A more holistic approach to resident needs, including those associated with privacy and sexuality, was lacking (Activity 8.1). Most staff time was spent on tasks related to residents' hygiene, nutrition, safety, and rest. Because sexuality has historically not been included in care planning for older adults, long-term care environments have not been designed in ways that are conducive to the fulfillment of sexual needs or that afford resident privacy.

REGULATIONS THAT DEFINE PRIVACY

As discussed in Chapter 3, nursing home staff and administration must comply with federal regulations and guidelines issued by the Centers for Medicare and Medicaid Services (CMS) that direct the way care should be delivered. This section highlights federal guidelines that address resident privacy in the long-term care environment. Each home must also be aware of state mandates that may add further instruction.

While nursing homes currently must comply with more rules and regulations than any other industries, save nuclear power, no regulations have addressed resident sexuality, and it appears unlikely that any new regulations will be created to govern the right of sexual expression, specifically as it relates to resident privacy. CMS has, however, issued several F-Tag regulations (short for

Nursing home residents have a right to personal privacy, including with respect to accommodations, medical treatment, written communications, personal care, visits, and meetings of family and resident groups. Residents have the right to privacy and to have their needs met, as long as those rights do not infringe on other residents' needs and rights. "Right to personal privacy" means that the resident has the right to privacy with whomever the resident wishes to be private and that this privacy should include full visual, and, to the extent desired, for visits or other activities, auditory privacy. Private space may be created flexibly and need not be dedicated solely for visitation purposes. (F-Tag 164 (483.10 (e)), Privacy and Confidentiality of Personal and Clinical Records)

"Federal Tags"), with accompanying Interpretive Guidelines, to assist long-term care facilities when addressing issues of resident privacy. The issue of privacy directly impacts resident sexuality.

The right to personal privacy, as defined by F-Tag 164 (483.10 (e)), Privacy and Confidentiality of Personal and Clinical Records, means that the resident has the right to privacy with whomever the resident wishes to be private and that this privacy should include full visual, and, to the extent desired, for visits or other activities, auditory privacy. Private space may be created flexibly and need not be dedicated solely for visitation purposes. (F-Tag 164 (483.10(e)), CMS Interpretive Guidelines)

F-Tag 454 (483.70 (d)), Physical Environment, defines privacy within the resident's room. It states that resident rooms must be "designed and equipped for adequate nursing care, comfort, and privacy of residents." F-Tag 460, Full Visual Privacy, requires room designs (e.g., ceiling-suspended curtains) that ensure the full visual privacy of residents. According to the CMS Interpretive Guidelines, full visual privacy means that

> residents have a means of completely withdrawing from public view while occupying their bed (e.g., curtain, moveable screens, private room). The guidelines do not intend to limit the provisions of privacy to solely one or more curtains, movable screens or a private room. Facility operators are free to use other means to provide full visual privacy, with those means varying according to the needs and requests of residents. (F-Tag 460 (483.70(d)(1)(iv), CMS Interpretive Guidelines)

With the exception of the explicit requirement for privacy curtains in all initially certified nursing homes (see §483.70(d)(1)(v)), facilities are free to innovate in designing care environments that ensure privacy for their residents. This may, but need not, be through the provision of a private room.

The right to privacy extends to visits from family members, friends, and other visitors. A facility cannot subject immediate family or other relatives or friends to visiting hour limitations or other restrictions not imposed by the resident. Likewise, facilities must provide 24-hour access to individuals who are not immediate relatives and who are visiting with the consent of the resident. These visitors are subject to "reasonable restrictions," according to the regulatory language, as well as the resident's right to deny or withdraw consent to visit at any time. Reasonable restrictions are those imposed by a facility to protect the security of all residents, such as keeping the home locked at night and denying access or providing limited and supervised access to a visitor who has abused, exploited, or coerced a resident; has committed criminal acts such as theft; or who has been inebriated and disruptive during past visits. If a resident's visitation rights infringe upon the rights of other residents, a facility may change the location of visits to assist in care giving or to protect the needs and privacy of other residents (e.g., late evening family visits that prevent the resident's roommate from sleeping).

The privacy considerations defined and regulated by CMS leave the door open for states to develop their own privacy policies related to the care environment to protect the right of residents to express themselves sexually (Activity 8.2).

PRIVATE VERSUS PUBLIC SPACE

When initially designing a building type, architects and designers typically base their plans on the needs of those who will be using the space. While there are many different types of nursing home buildings across the United States, most were designed around the assumptions of health care delivery systems during the industrial era, and as a consequence, tend to be rigid in their use. They do not lend themselves to easily accommodating human interactions outside the realm of health care delivery. If we consider what the seniors of today expect of nursing homes (care environments that address their holistic needs, not just their medical needs), we see that past assumptions need to change.

Nursing home residents often live for a significant number of years within the walls of a building that was conceived to be an institution, not a home. And because it is a home, barriers to sexual expression that exist in the care settings must be identified and addressed. When considering the role of the physical environment in supporting intimacy, it is important to consider the setting as a whole. Starting from the general layout of a typical institutional building to the type of furniture a nursing home provides, intimate relationships are impacted by the physical elements of spaces.

HOME AS A PLACE OF INTIMATE RELATIONSHIPS

The word *home* is often associated with a place that is central to an individual's life. Reflecting on the meaning of home may trigger images of a structure, or more importantly memories of relationships that were a part of the experience of home. The significance of home extends beyond memories and simple imagery. Homes are territories used to establish boundaries between members of a family and the outside world. They also guard privacy and the nature and intimacy of family activities. Some of us have been fortunate enough to have a place to call home all of our lives. The behaviors associated with family and home have been a part of our identity since before we could walk and talk. We learned to respect the privacy of the people with whom we lived by interacting with them and by relating certain behaviors to different spaces in the home environment. It may have been so long ago since these early lessons were learned, however, that their significance may now seem trivial. We respond intuitively, usually without much conscious thought, about how spaces relate to and affect our activities and behaviors.

Home designs commonly provide at least four basic levels of privacy through designation of specific rooms as well as the location and type of access—public, semipublic, private, and semiprivate. Public domains connect people to the broader community, such as picking up the mail and sitting on the front porch. Semipublic spaces are designated for activities such as housekeeping, cooking, eating, and general forms of recreation (watching the television or working on a hobby). Semipublic spaces might be provided as quiet rooms, family dining rooms, or living rooms—places that are specifically designated as family visiting areas. Depending on individual situations or specific features of a space, these may also be rooms or even transitional spaces where a guest can be invited to interact. Semiprivate spaces are often associated with areas where we interact with family members in loosely structured ways. These spaces are still environments where receiving guests is not a formal activity, and the nature of these spaces and their relationship to other spaces allow users to feel at ease. These areas may also provide space for work that does not invite guests, such as a laundry room or a home office. The most private activities, sleeping, bathing, grooming, toileting, and intimate sexual activity, take place in the private domains of a home (bedrooms and bathrooms).

Each home is unique in its layout and assignment of spaces depending on family needs, but there is usually a mix of public and private spaces. Where guests are greeted and included in activities is also fairly consistent; there are rooms that feel welcoming, and rooms that guests would not enter without expressed permission. The physical features of space (e.g., walls and doors) and the placement of rooms distinguish private areas from other public areas, as do social norms of behavior. Nursing homes must have these principles in mind when designing environments for residents to honor privacy.

CHANGING THE CULTURE OF PRIVACY IN THE NURSING HOME ENVIRONMENT

Nursing home designs typically do not provide clear boundaries between public and private spaces and, therefore, significantly reduce the levels of privacy that can be achieved. As mentioned earlier, many nursing home designs mimic those of hospitals, with a public corridor and hallway that runs directly from a space that is considered the most private in a residential home—the bedroom (Figure 8.1). The original designs of long-term care settings did not take into account the intimacies of home life and, therefore, the experience of privacy has often felt shallow.

Changing the culture of privacy in nursing homes involves a shift away from an institutional experience for older adults to a residential one that supports personal relationships. An important first step to begin this process is to explore how

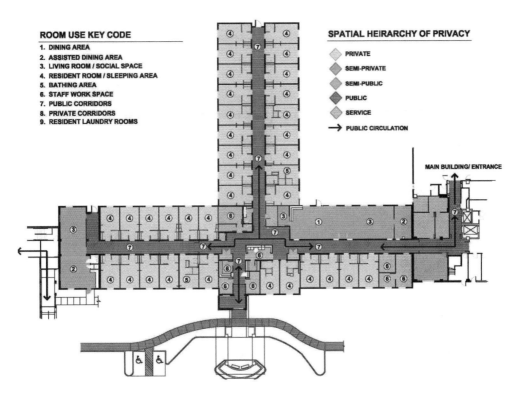

ROOM USE KEY CODE

1. DINING AREA
2. ASSISTED DINING AREA
3. LIVING ROOM / SOCIAL SPACE
4. RESIDENT ROOM / SLEEPING AREA
5. BATHING AREA
6. STAFF WORK SPACE
7. PUBLIC CORRIDORS
8. PRIVATE CORRIDORS
9. RESIDENT LAUNDRY ROOMS

SPATIAL HEIRARCHY OF PRIVACY

PRIVATE
SEMI-PRIVATE
SEMI-PUBLIC
PUBLIC
SERVICE
→ PUBLIC CIRCULATION

MAIN BUILDING/ ENTRANCE

Figure 8.1 Spatial zones of a typical nursing home.

the nursing home environment can better support privacy and intimacy. Seemingly trivial details regarding space must be focused on to capture the fundamental essence of what *home* means to older adults and to understand how spaces can be formed and arranged to support privacy and intimacy, including sexuality.

By their design, nursing homes are larger than private homes, bringing more individuals together than most people would normally experience in their daily living situations. The ability to control access to individual residents, therefore, may become a seemingly impossible task as access to the collective whole often overrides the needs of individual residents and couples. If staff and administrators consider the context of privacy as it relates to the control of access, however, they can focus on the importance of creating spaces that afford the appropriate levels of privacy to support personal relationships within the setting. This requires scrutinizing the rooms in a facility and the patterns of movement between these rooms. For example, in residential home designs, bedrooms typically are not placed by the front door, and people typically do not socialize or invite guests into their bedrooms. Such is not the case in nursing home environments, where the arrangement of spaces often places private bedroom areas adjacent to public areas, such as common hallways and nurses' stations where visitors to the building come and go (Figure 8.2).

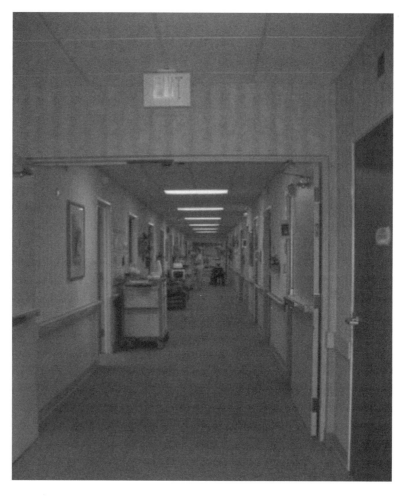

Figure 8.2 View down public hallway in a nursing home setting.

Federal regulations may mandate standards for basic human dignity and privacy (e.g., staff should knock, close the door); however, if the spaces of the care environment are not designed to respect the privacy of residents, then an essential feature of home is lost.

Reclaiming the Intimacy of Home

Facilities that have effectively created an experience of home have paid attention to the arrangement of spaces and the sequential nature of circulation between rooms that should have various levels of privacy (Figure 8.3). Cues from features in the built environment can send a powerful message to staff, visitors, and also residents. For example, a front door implies that anyone, including family, should request permission to enter.

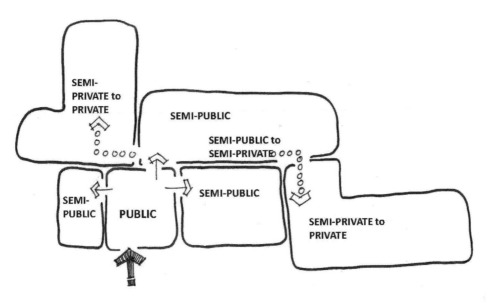

Figure 8.3 A public to private continuum.

Inside the home, walls and doors can also provide privacy cues. Hallways are often underappreciated features of residential homes. These spaces signal to guests where and where not to go and control access to more private areas. In some long-term care settings, for example, hallways have been identified as the "enemy" and the designs have focused on eliminating them by circling resident bedrooms around social areas. While residents may be able to step right outside their bedroom door to get a seat at the dining table, they are also going to be in the center of every social activity that takes place. A resident's ability to control access to him- or herself has been sacrificed for the sake of eliminating any significant circulation route and to get residents to common areas quickly and efficiently.

There is no easy fix. The challenge in modifying institutional hallways involves both length and public access. If planned strategically, however, hallways can be used as a buffer zone between private and public spaces and can send a very clear signal about the nature of access to the spaces along the hallways and beyond. As a result, the potential to create a variety of privacy levels can increase dramatically (Figure 8.4).

Personal Spaces—Private versus Shared Rooms

Another challenge for many nursing homes is the resident room itself (Figures 8.5 and 8.6). Again, following a medical model of architecture, many nursing homes still financially depend on rooms for two residents. Room design standards for regulatory compliance can date back to guidelines from the 1970s.

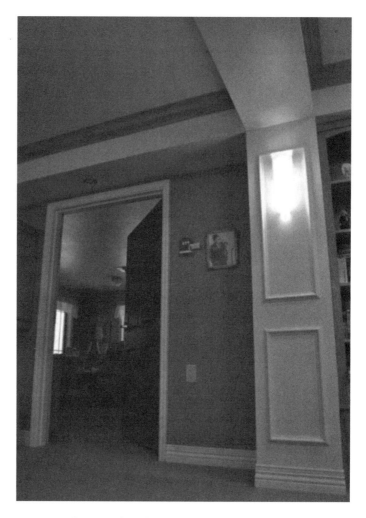

Figure 8.4   View into resident room from the corridor.

Furthermore, nursing home architecture of the past 50 years has focused on meeting regulatory standards and providing the appropriate support for staff to deliver care within a limited definition of applicable solutions to achieve required outcomes.

These standards outline minimum square footages required in most rooms of a facility, including the minimum space requirements for private and shared resident sleeping areas. Some current design concepts have identified ways to better respect privacy and support autonomy through more single-occupancy room and space options. Little evidence, however, has shown that nursing homes are modifying space standards to create personal spaces. The only significant changes in space standards for resident rooms have occurred as a result of the passage of the Americans with Disabilities Act (ADA) in 1990 and the implementation of the ADA Accessibility Guidelines (ADAAG) for all new construction (construction,

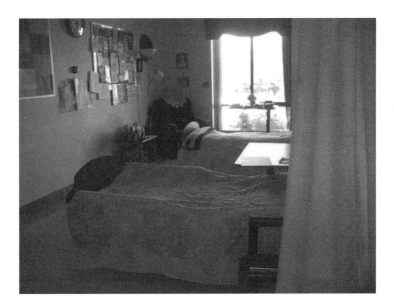

Figure 8.5 Side-by-side bed configuration in a shared room.

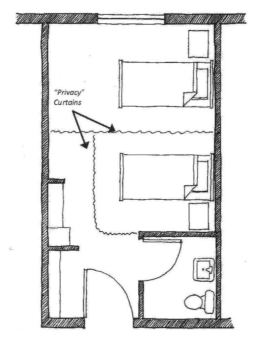

Figure 8.6 Side-by-side bed configuration in a shared room.

modification or alterations) (ADA, 1991). For example, bathrooms for resident rooms in skilled nursing facilities must allow for a turning radius of 5 feet in diameter. Existing facilities have often been permitted to maintain smaller space standards until they can undergo significant remodeling.

Facilities that have adopted new space standards have also incorporated fixed interior features that provide a more defined separation between two sides of a room (Figures 8.7 and 8.8). These types of rooms use a full-height wall partition that gives more visual and auditory privacy as well as another location for the arrangement of furniture.

Functional Bedroom Space

Resident bedroom designs should be considered in terms of both quantity of space and quality of the spatial arrangement in providing opportunities for resident autonomy and privacy. Square footage dictates the quantity of bedroom furniture that can be placed in a room (Figure 8.9). Design considerations cannot simply stop at the overall quantity of space, but should also focus on the quality of space and a resident's ability to place personal possessions within the space (usable space). General usable area can be calculated by subtracting the overall total area needed for doors to swing, entry hallways, or parts of the room that are not usable for a piece of furniture. Other considerations should include cross-over space and circulation in relation to a roommate's personal area if the room is shared.

Furnishings and Features
that Support or Impede Intimacy

Within private spaces, the bed plays a significant role in supporting privacy and intimacy. Sleep patterns may change later in life and some married couples find that sleeping apart leads to better sleep. This sleeping arrangement may very well be continued when a couple moves into a long-term care facility. For a couple to have two twin beds in their room, however, could pose an issue regarding sexual intimacy. Because they are designed for a single individual, a twin (or single) bed would not allow enough space for a couple to share physical intimacy. And sex is not sleep; it is a physical activity that is benefited by having some space to maneuver and adjust. As discussed previously, the general floor space of the sleeping area dictates the type and size of furniture the room can accommodate. Rooms for couples require floor space for either two single or one double bed. If a couple move into a nursing home together and single beds are necessary for sleep or medical considerations, the placement of other furnishings in relation to the beds may support privacy and intimacy. For example, a comfortable chair next to the bed would support physical contact (holding hands) and comfort between individuals, one or both of whom may have functional mobility limitations (Figure 8.10).

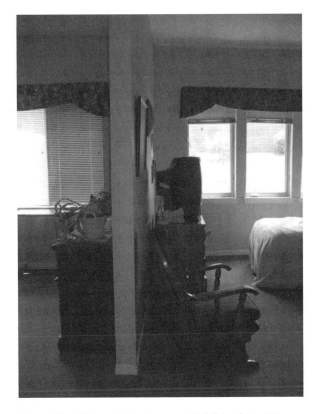

Figure 8.7 Enhanced shared room with full height partition.

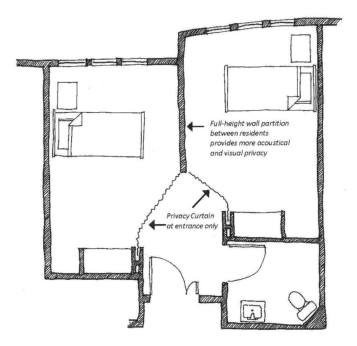

Figure 8.8 Enhanced shared room with full height partition.

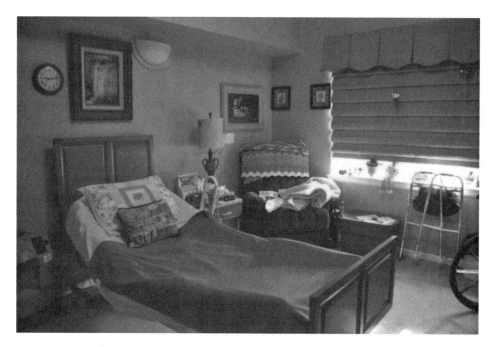

Figure 8.9 A resident room should provide flexibility in bed size and placement.

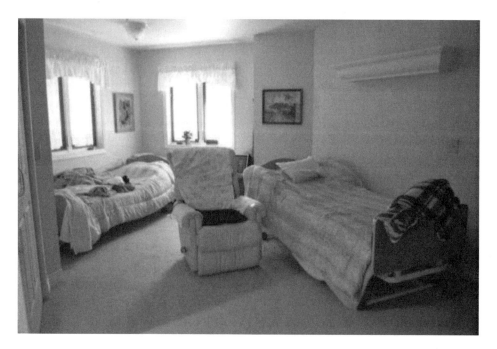

Figure 8.10 Furniture placed close to a bed to support physical contact and comfort between couples.

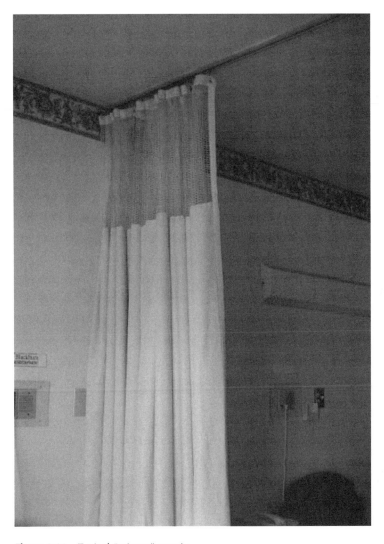

Figure 8.11 Typical "privacy" curtain.

Other features of the room also impact the type of privacy experienced in residents' bedroom space. For shared rooms, the minimum regulatory standard of separation between residents is a privacy curtain that is suspended from a ceiling track (Figure 8.11). The National Fire Protection Association Life Safety Code requires that the top 18 inches of the curtain be a mesh weave that will permit the penetration of fire suppression agents dispersed from sprinkler heads in the event of a fire. The consequence, however, is that there is little to any acoustical barrier with a ceiling-suspended curtain. Personal conversations cannot be adequately shielded, and if one roommate is trying to share a private moment with a lover, the other will likely feel obligated to leave the room.

The Balance between Space and Policy

Any changes to the built environment to support privacy and intimacy will be ineffective unless there are also changes to a nursing home's policies. Space standards and the program of care are so interrelated that if both are not considered together, their potential effectiveness is compromised. The planned program of care can outline activities and types of experiences desired for residents and staff, but the spaces to support the activities have to be put into place in order for the experiences to be realized. It means changing established patterns of schedules and procedures.

Long-term care facilities are complicated entities. There are construction standards and regulations in place for the protection of residents and staff. Most architects and designers are far removed from the daily activities of long-term care facilities. Even those firms that have broad experience designing long-term care facilities may not have a solid sense of what it means to design spaces that provide a level of privacy that supports intimacy. In essence the multiple layers of support for privacy are the "union" of a program of care and the right building design. The activities that will take place in the home should be defined, and the environment should be supportive of those patterns of life.

ORGANIZATIONAL AND RESIDENT PERSPECTIVES ON PRIVATE SPACES

Some of the most useful studies of private versus shared spaces have evaluated their psychosocial outcomes, typically by measuring satisfaction levels among residents. An AARP survey found that people over the age of 50 preferred a private room by a ratio of 20 to 1 (Baugh, 1996). Factors for this preference included greater privacy (for self and for engaging with others), more control (over lifestyle and environment), and having felt uncomfortable after being forced to be an "unwilling observer" to others in a shared room. These results mirror earlier findings by Lawton and Bader (1970), who found the preference for a private room to be 92% of community dwelling individuals and 85%–95% of nursing home residents who were living in private rooms.

In a fascinating study from Japan (Terakawa, 2004), nursing home residents were followed as they moved from a traditional nursing home with shared rooms to one with private rooms. Residents were interviewed prior to the move, 1 month after the move, and 8 months later. All residents, even those who did not expect to like having a private room, were completely positive about the change at 8 months. This result is interesting because the Japanese culture is traditionally more communally focused. The authors speculated that resident opinions about satisfaction with having a shared room may have been based on being reasonably satisfied with current living conditions and not on having had experience with both private and semi-private rooms.

Much of the research from hospital settings has shown that patients feel they have better visits when in private rooms (Kaldenburg, 1999; Ulrich & Zimring, 2004). Patients also report feeling more in control, especially regarding the radio or television, heating or cooling, opening or closing curtains or doors, and personalizing and decorating the room.

The type of space also affects residents' ability to establish and maintain social bonds, which are essential to overall well-being as people grow older. It would seem that close ties could develop between roommates in long-term care. One study, however, found that only 22% of roommates had strong or positive emotional bonds with their roommate, while another 78% had moderate or weak bonds (Bitzan, 1998). Even the strong bonders did not enjoy spending time with their roommate, did not perceive their roommate to be sensitive to their needs, and said they got along best when they kept their feelings and activities to themselves.

Clinical evidence has shown that the quality of sleep improves for residents in private rooms (Schnelle, Alexxi, Al-Sameeai, Fricker, & Ouslander, 1999). The improvement primarily stems from staff not having to enter a room at night to care for a roommate. Infection control also improves with private rooms (Zimmerman, Gruber-Baldini, Hebel, Sloane, & Magaziner, 2002). There is mixed evidence about falls (Chaudhury, Mahmood, & Valente, 2005). Some anecdotal reports from nurses suggest that roommates can help prevent falls by reminding each other not to take risks. Other reports, however, suggest that either there is no difference in the rate of falls or that falls are reduced with single rooms.

With all the evidence pointing to the benefits of private rooms in nursing homes, it would seem that there would be more of them available. To understand better why this is not the case, it is important to examine the organizational factors that come into play.

Calkins and Cassella (2007) assessed private rooms based on three factors: (1) organizational, including design, capital costs for construction, and building operation; (2) operational, including staffing, marketing or maintaining census, and time spent managing residents; and (3) resident, including psychosocial outcomes (well-being, satisfaction) and clinical issues (sleep, falls, infections). Their findings regarding resident outcomes were similar to those of previous studies. Staff also reported in focus groups a reduced need for psychotropic medications, fewer medical errors, and less behavioral problems with residents in private rooms.

Anecdotal evidence regarding operational factors suggests problems with trying to market shared rooms. Calkins and Cassella (2007) argued that nursing homes lose income trying to market shared rooms. Private rooms, on the other hand, generally have long wait lists and, therefore, are more consistent sources of revenue. Some retirement communities may lose residents if the residents perceive they will not be able to have a private room should the need arise.

For issues related to staff, problems arise in maintaining resident confidentiality regarding medications (the need to discuss their use in the presence of a roommate). Nurses also judged private rooms as requiring further walking distances (Chaudhury, Mahmood, & Valente, 2004). Higher costs result from the amount of time staff spend on managing roommate conflicts. Some nurses report spending hours per day trying to soothe upset residents. If conflicts are not resolved, additional hours must be used to relocate a resident and to clean and prepare a room for the next roommate. Sometimes few rooms are available for moves, which can cause a time- and cost-consuming domino effect.

Calkins and Cassella (2007) prepared a cost analysis that showed that a home could recoup the cost of private rooms within less than 2 years. Furthermore, that time could be reduced if a home consistently has empty beds available.

This type of research is critical to the leaders in long-term care housing. Organizations can only implement design considerations to improve resident well-being, staff outcomes, and the bottom line if they can afford to stay open. Administrators must have clear operational guidance when factoring in considerations regarding private spaces.

RESIDENT PRIVACY RELATED TO VISITS

As discussed earlier, federal and state guidelines mandate that nursing homes provide privacy and dignity for residents. While no federal or state regulations attempt to address sexuality explicitly, most state regulators have suggested that issues related to sexuality fall under the more general resident right guidelines related to visits and privacy (Nursing Home Regulations Plus, 2011).

Federal guidelines address resident rights to privacy for visits by various persons. Eighteen States (Alaska, Colorado, Delaware, Idaho, Illinois, Iowa, Kentucky, Michigan, Mississippi, Missouri, New Jersey, New Mexico, North Dakota, Rhode Island, South Carolina, Virginia, and Wisconsin) consider the issue of shared rooms specifically for spouses living in a nursing home or for conjugal visits. Each of these states, with the exception of Colorado, discuss the issue in terms of marital status. Colorado recognizes the right of nursing home residents to "private consensual activity" without including statements about marital relationships.

Most state regulations use language that suggests privacy must be provided for spousal visits; only Michigan, however, spells out what privacy should entail: A married nursing home resident "is entitled to meet privately with his or her spouse in a room that ensures privacy." This may imply, but it is not necessarily interpreted to mean, that the couple can lock the door from the inside.

Federal regulations mandating privacy and confidentiality for residents include privacy for visits but add that this does not require the facility to provide private rooms for residents. Yet without private rooms it is hard to fulfill privacy rights related to conjugal visits and other sexual activity, or even "immediate access" to visitors of the resident's choice (Sidebar 8.1).

Only four states use language suggesting that intimate relationships might be with someone other than a spouse (Colorado, New Jersey, Rhode Island, Vermont). "Private and intimate physical and social interaction with other people," "spouse or other partner," and "reciprocal beneficiaries" are phrasings used by these states. Colorado clearly states the right to "consensual sexual activity" with no marital or medical restrictions. These four state statutes have allowed room for the possibility of sexual relationships between persons of the same gender or unmarried persons. It is interesting to note that no state regulations or guidelines make reference to common-law spouses (Activity 8.3).

STAFFING PRACTICES THAT CAN SUPPORT RESIDENT PRIVACY

In long-term care the provision of private rooms or private spaces is not enough to assure privacy for resident sexual expression. Staff practices can also play a role in supporting resident privacy in the care environment.

There are several steps that staff can take to ensure the privacy of those in their care. Always waiting for permission to enter a room after knocking is one important way of honoring residents' need to control their environment. Staff should also choose to discuss sensitive information (medications, medical treatments) when other persons (roommate, visitors) are not present. Regarding resident sexuality, staff may choose to help residents to rent a hotel room for the night, move beds together or permit the use of a double bed, hang do-not-disturb signs, or make other accommodations to provide privacy for sexual activities. It may also be possible to move a resident's bed so it is not visible from the door, especially if a room is off a public corridor.

"Visiting Room" Guidelines

These guidelines were established to accommodate the rights of residents who wish to have overnight visitors. The facility recognizes the rights of residents to privacy and confidentiality. The right to privacy extends to the right to meet in private with others, including full visual and auditory privacy.

All visitors are to be treated as guests who have entered the home of a loved one. Reasonable accommodations, staff attitudes, and dignity will be provided to guests while they are visiting.

The visiting room may be used by two consenting residents, or by a resident who has a guest from the community.

The nursing facility is required to provide care and services to a resident to meet the resident's highest practicable physical, mental, and psychosocial well-being. This facility provides for overnight and daytime private visits for residents and guests under the following guidelines.

VISITING ROOM

Eligibility for use of the visiting room.   Residents may invite guests from outside the facility to stay in the visiting room for designated nights. Two consenting residents may request the use of the visiting room.

Reserving the visiting room.   The visiting room is available to residents and their guests. The room may be available on short notice by contacting the Social Services director. In the event a conflict exists, a schedule will be established and reservations will be taken in advance. The Social Services director will be responsible for maintaining the list and reminding visitors of their reservations.

Orientation for outside overnight visitors.   Visitors who are not residents of the facility and staying in the visiting room must be oriented to the facility regulations and safety guidelines, which include the following:

- *Call light.* Demonstrate the use of the call light to the visitor. Explain the purpose of the light, expected time staff will need to respond to the light, and the tasks staff can and cannot complete.

Sidebar 8.1 (continued)

- *Meals.* Explain the meal arrangements, hours, diet restrictions, and any cost associated with meals provided by the facility. Visitors may bring meals into the facility provided this does not conflict with physician orders for the resident. Alcoholic beverages may be brought into the facility and served to the resident with physician's consent.

- *Assistance from staff.* Visitors must be oriented to the roles staff provide in the facility. Staff must continue to provide care for the resident as indicated on the Care Plan and physician orders. Staff may not request the visitor provide care usually assigned to be delivered by professional staff in the facility.

- *Emergency orientation.* Orient visitors to emergency exits, fire alarms, wander guard alarms, and emergency procedures. In the event an emergency occurs while the visitor is on the premises, it is the responsibility of the visitor to comply with instructions provided by facility staff.

- *Medical emergency.* In the event of an emergency for the visitor, staff will call 911 and provide first aid until emergency responders arrive to the facility.

- *Confidentiality.* Staff are to request that visitors respect the confidentiality of other residents and that they refrain from sharing observed care delivered to other residents.

- *Staff provision of care.* Staff are required to provide care normally provided to the resident. Regularly scheduled medications, clothing changes, dressing changes, and ordered procedures must be provided per physician orders and as indicated on the Care Plan.

Fees. Fees to use the visiting room are restricted to the cost of meals.

Meals. Fees normally applied to visitors' meals will apply to all meals served to the visitor. Visitors are to be informed in advance of expected costs associated with meals. The guest will be oriented to the menu for meals prepared by facility staff.

(continued on next page)

Sidebar 8.1 (continued)

Showering facilities.   Orient the visitor to the shower area and bathroom facilities and provide appropriate linens. If the visitor requests soap, shampoo, and toothpaste, every effort will be made to accommodate those requests.

Arrival and departure time for overnight visitors.   The facility may request that the visitor arrive during hours when staff can be most accommodating. Staff may request a check-out time that provides ample opportunity for room cleaning. Arrival and departure times may be reflective of hotel check-in and check-out times (e.g., 3:00 check-in time and 12:00 noon check-out time).

Daytime hours.   The visiting room must be made available during regular visiting hours to accommodate the visitors who choose not to stay during the overnight hours. Special hours can be arranged through the Social Services Department.

Locking door.   The visiting room has a door with a lock that can be locked from inside the room. Staff are to retain a key and may use it in the event of an emergency.

Respect, dignity, and confidentiality.   As with all residents, utmost attention must be given to dignity, privacy, and confidentiality. At no time will staff be permitted to gossip, tease, or make derogatory comments about residents who use the visiting room, or use the visiting room as reward or punishment.

Furnishings.   The visiting room is designed to accommodate residents and their overnight guests. Every effort will be made to create comfortable surroundings. The facility will provide all necessary linens, resident care items, and reasonable special requests.

Room cleaning.   Facility staff are responsible for cleaning the room before and after use by guests. Clean linens, floors, shower areas, and furnishings will be provided for each guest.

Follow-up.   At the conclusion of the visit, guests will be invited to return, whether by written correspondence or verbally.

Sidebar 8.1 (continued)

There are no regulations suggesting that a room should be provided for conjugal visits for residents who do not have a private room. Most homes cannot afford to give up a resident room for a dedicated conjugal visit room, but some have made the following compromises:

- Schedule visits when the other roommate is getting her hair done or attending an activity.

- Help the couple to make arrangements at a hotel. This has been done for special occasions like anniversaries or birthdays.

- Make an unoccupied room available for one night.

- Find ways to make resident rooms more private (i.e., wait for response after knocking and before entering a room).

- Add locks on the inside of a room.

- Accommodate family caregivers. One nursing home allows caregiving spouses to stay in the assisted living room with their mate for an additional $500 per month in rent. They usually maintain a primary residence in the community, and this keeps the residents connected with their spouses while also giving them the freedom they may need.

- Consider all possibilities, including whether this is appropriate for nonmarried couples and more casual relationships.

Source: Guidelines on pages 202–204 were prepared by Carol Marshall, M.A., health care consultant. Reprinted with permission. Guidelines on page 205 regarding conjugal visits were prepared by the author (Gayle Appel Doll).

DISCUSSION

Return to the story at the beginning of the chapter. What would you do? Have a conversation with your co-workers about this incident and then write out a plan of action to address it. How can both the residents' and family members' privacy and dignity and the ability to control situations be honored?

SUMMARY

Nursing homes were initially designed to be efficient in providing care, with little or no consideration for the privacy of residents. Many nursing home organizations are now recognizing this and trying to modify their environment to provide a more holistic approach to caregiving that includes acknowledging and respecting the privacy needs of residents. Staff practices can also be modified to support and protect the privacy of residents. While assisted living homes provide better opportunities for privacy because of the provision of private rooms, staff actions may limit privacy and opportunities for sexual expression.

REFERENCES

Americans with Disabilities Act: Accessibility Guidelines for Buildings and Facilities. (1991). Washington, D.C.: U. S. Architectural and Transportation Barriers Compliance Board.

Baugh, T. (1996). *Shared housing focus groups.* Washington, DC: American Association of Retired Persons.

Bauer, M. (1999). Their only privacy is between their sheets: Privacy and sexuality of elderly nursing home residents. *Journal of Gerontological Nursing, 25*(8), 37–41.

Bitzan, J. (1998). Emotional bondedness and subjective well-being between nursing home residents. *Journal of Gerontological Nursing, 24*, 8–15.

Calkins, M., & Cassella, C. (2007). Exploring the cost and value of private versus shared bedrooms in nursing homes. *The Gerontologist, 47*, 168–183.

Chaudhury, H., Mahmood, A., & Valente, M. (2004). *Nurses' perceptions of single versus multi-occupancy rooms in acute care environments: An exploratory comparative assessment.* Vancouver, BC: Simon Frasier University.

Chaudhury, H., Mahmood, A., & Valente, M. (2005). Advantages and disadvantages of single-versus multiple-occupancy rooms in acute care environments. *Environment and Behavior, 20*, 1–27.

Kaldenberg, D. (1999). The influence of having a roommate on patient satisfaction. *The Satisfaction Monitor, 3–4.*

Lawton, M., & Bader, J. (1970). Wish for privacy by young and old. *Journal of Gerontology, 25*(1), 48–54.

Nursing Home Regulations Plus. (2011). Retrieved from http://www.sph.umn.edu/hpm/nhregsplus/federal_regulations.htm.

Schnelle, J. F., Alessi, C. A., Al-Samarrai, N. R., Fricker, R. D., & Ouslander, J. G. (1999). The nursing home at night: Effects of an intervention on noise, light, and sleep. *Journal of the American Geriatric Society, 47*, 430–438.

Terakawa, Y. (2004, June). The relationship between environment and behavior at the institutional setting for the elderly. Paper presented at the annual conference of the Environmental Design Research Association, Albuquerque, NM.

Ulrich, R., & Zimring, C. (2004). *The Role of the Physical Environment in the Hospital of the 21st Century: A Once in a Lifetime Opportunity.* Concord, CA: Center for Health Design.

Zimmerman, S., Gruber-Baldini, A., Hebel, J., Sloane, P., & Magaziner, J. (2002). Nursing home facility risk factors for infection and hospitalization: Importance of registered nurse turnover, administration and social factors. *Journal of the American Geriatrics Society, 50*, 1987–1995.

Privacy in the Home

Staff and resident perceptions of privacy may vary. One way to find out if this is true in your home is to give disposable cameras to staff and residents and ask them to take pictures of the places in the home that they would go to if they wanted privacy. Compare the pictures. Bring residents and staff together to talk about the results.

Many homes have added private living or dining rooms to their facilities so that residents may have areas for private conversations. Research has shown, however, that residents use these rooms very little (Calkins & Cassella, 2007). Some homes may add them more as a marketing feature to impress families and less with the residents' privacy needs in mind.

Sexuality and Long-Term Care: Understanding and Supporting the Needs of Older Adults, by Gayle Appel Doll
(Copyright 2012, by Health Professions Press, Inc.)

What's Your Policy?

Review your state regulations and guidelines regarding privacy. Do they do enough to protect residents' ability to express themselves sexually? If not, suggest ways they can be improved.

Policy Implications

Consider how your home could take steps to improve privacy in the care environment to support intimate relationships. If a conjugal or visit room is not a reasonable option, what other opportunities might be afforded?

9

Health and Sexuality

OBJECTIVES

- Describe the physiological changes that occur with age that may affect sexual expression
- List the disease and health problems that can interfere with sexual health
- Describe assessments for sexual health
- Identify interventions to maintain or restore sexual health
- Examine the prevalence of sexually transmitted disease in aging populations
- Discuss education strategies for safer sexual activity

he nurses at Oakdale Heights assisted living were having a problem with Charlie. His doctor had prescribed medication for hypertension, but after several weeks of improvement in his blood pressure, it began to rise again. After some very persistent questioning, Charlie admitted that he had stopped taking his medication because it had kept him from "working down there."

PHYSIOLOGICAL CHANGES WITH AGE THAT AFFECT SEXUALITY

Older adults report sexual desire but decreased sexual activity as they age. Some of this reduction is due to physiological changes associated with growing older. In females these changes include loss of vaginal elasticity and lubrication and slowed response time. Older women remain capable of achieving intense and multiple orgasms, and for some women sex is more enjoyable after menopause because of the cessation of fertility. This presupposes that birth control is no longer needed. For protection from sexually transmitted diseases (STDs), however, older women should insist that their partners wear a condom. Researchers have found that attitudes about sex, personal values, and accessibility of partners are more predictive of sexual activity in women than physiological changes (Delamater & Moorman, 2007).

Older men experience reductions in sexual desire, less firm erections, delay in achieving an erection, a decrease in penile sensitivity, and delayed orgasm. Some men experiencing these changes may not know that they are normal and may suspect impotence. Psychological and medical interventions can be used to overcome these problems. One sexual advantage for older men is that they can maintain an erection much longer than younger men.

Most older adults living in long-term care have had little to no sexual education and do not discuss sexual activity with friends, family, or health care providers. They may also not be aware of what physiological changes related to aging that affect sexual function are normal and what changes are not normal (are pathological or due to a disease process). Sex education can help them to understand these changes (Activity 9.1). Older Americans, for example, are the fastest-growing demographic to be infected with the human immunodeficiency virus (HIV), which causes acquired immunodeficiency syndrome (AIDS). The factors associated with high risk include sexual contact with prostitutes, illicit drug use, and the failure to use condoms. This population is also the least likely to be targeted for prevention. Health care providers, probably assuming asexuality among older adults or because they are fearful of embarrassing an older person, often choose not to bring up the subject of protection against HIV infection.

DISEASES AND OTHER PATHOLOGICAL PROBLEMS

The diseases that affect sexual function include diabetes, hypertension, heart disease, incontinence, kidney disease, stroke, and neurological and cognitive disorders (dementia, Parkinson's disease, and so forth). For example, up to one-third of community-dwelling older adults and more than half of nursing home residents experience incontinence at least temporarily (Haleem, 2004). Although incontinence does not necessarily affect sexual function, it can affect a person's feelings of attractiveness and certainly can cause embarrassment in sexual situations. Many people are so embarrassed by this problem that they frequently fail to report it to a health professional. There are many ways to treat incontinence that could lead to a better sexual experience.

Medications taken to treat these diseases may also interfere with sexual function. In addition to the affect on sexual function, the disease state and medications may drain an older adult's energy levels, lessen sexual interest, and decrease feelings of attractiveness.

ASSESSING FOR SEXUAL HEALTH

One tool health care professionals can use to assess sexual health is Permission, Limited Information, Specific Suggestions, and Intensive Therapy (PLISSIT) (Wallace, 2008). This assessment model provides the following steps for gathering information from older adults:

1. *Permission.* Permission can be interpreted to mean either asking for permission to evaluate or giving the older person permission to discuss sexuality. "Would it be all right if I asked you some questions about how your medication has affected your sexual health?" Asking permission puts the resident in control. This question should be followed with a series of open-ended questions specific to sexual health: What concerns do you have? What changes have you had in your feelings about sexuality? The assessor might ask to have the resident's spouse or partner join the discussion.

2. *Limited information.* The health care professional should provide a resident with information about physiological changes related to aging that may affect sexuality.

3. *Specific suggestions.* Based on the resident's responses to open-ended questions the nurse or other health care professional makes suggestions for a plan of care.

4. *Intensive therapy.* Intensive therapy may be indicated for people with health problems beyond normal aging.

A protocol developed by Letvak and Schoder (1996) can be used to collect a resident's sexual history (Sidebar 9.1). As discussed in Chapters 6, the history can assist staff in assessing sexual behaviors that may be seen as inappropriate but may in fact be due to impaired judgment or impulse control stemming from a medical condition or medication. In the case of assessing a resident's sexual health, the increase in HIV infection and other STDs can be expressed as a justification for discussing his or her sexual history. Letvak and Schoder encourage those collecting the information to keep in mind that sexual activity may include body parts other

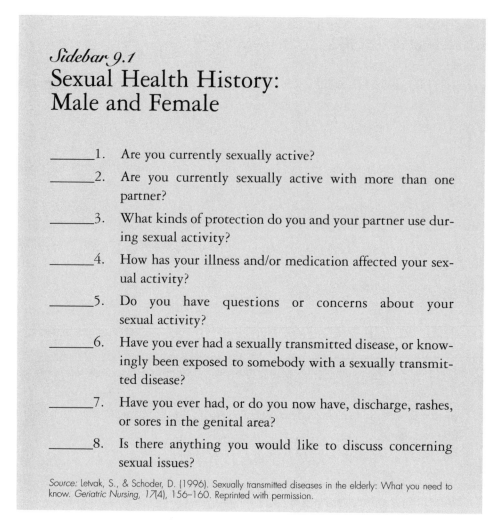

Sidebar 9.1

Sexual Health History:
Male and Female

_____1. Are you currently sexually active?

_____2. Are you currently sexually active with more than one partner?

_____3. What kinds of protection do you and your partner use during sexual activity?

_____4. How has your illness and/or medication affected your sexual activity?

_____5. Do you have questions or concerns about your sexual activity?

_____6. Have you ever had a sexually transmitted disease, or knowingly been exposed to somebody with a sexually transmitted disease?

_____7. Have you ever had, or do you now have, discharge, rashes, or sores in the genital area?

_____8. Is there anything you would like to discuss concerning sexual issues?

Source: Letvak, S., & Schoder, D. (1996). Sexually transmitted diseases in the elderly: What you need to know. *Geriatric Nursing, 17*(4), 156–160. Reprinted with permission.

than genitalia (mouth, anus), and that even older people engage in different types of sexual activity.

Because sexuality can be such a sensitive subject, staff may choose to wait to do this particular assessment until they have been able to establish trust with a new resident. If the sexual history is discussed during a health assessment, it should not be saved until the end because this may indicate to the resident that the person conducting the interview is uncomfortable with the subject (thereby making the resident feel uncomfortable). It is better to start with topics that are easy to discuss and then move on to more difficult ones. Open-ended questions provide more information than yes and no responses (e.g., What are your experiences with heterosexual and homosexual activities?). Beginning questions with a more global "Many people ask questions about . . ." may also help to ease some of the discomfort of these questions. A long-term care facility may also choose to create a form that residents can complete on their own.

INTERVENTIONS FOR MAINTAINING AND RESTORING SEXUAL HEALTH

Covington Heights nursing home had a new policy modeled after the Make-a-Wish Foundation. The staff were interviewing the residents to find out what activities they desired that the home could arrange for. They had already made a trip to the local casino with a busload of residents. Two other residents had requested an airplane ride and a ride on a Harley motorcycle. Staff began to have second thoughts about the new practice when Arnold requested a night with a female staff member. After some prodding, Arnold modified his request to a staff wet T-shirt contest. One of the staff members took the request to the administrator for advice. He asked staff members to loan him T-shirts from home. He hosed them down and hung them in the dining room during dinner. The residents were asked to vote for their favorite wet shirt. There was no report about how Arnold felt about the activity. One can hope that he at least retained his sense of humor.

Nursing homes are expected to create "normal" living environments, which would include attention to all the usual rhythms of life, including sexual activity. In a perfect world residents would have access to private spaces as well as condoms and vaginal lubricants. Male residents would be screened for erectile dysfunction and offered consultation and performance-enhancing drugs. Private spaces would be made available for the least disruptive sexual activity—masturbation. Female residents would be able to purchase vibrators and dildos, and staff would be trained to be respectful of these needs.

Should staff have to provide for these needs? Should they address residents' needs proactively or just when requested? Should staff have to provide explicit materials, such as pornographic videos and and magazines? Should they be expected to obtain these materials for residents? A liberal view of the long-term care environment would include sexual health and quality of life in supporting resident well-being and dignity. These questions and possible staff interventions need to be addressed within the context of individual nursing home policies because they have not, and likely will not, be addressed within federal and state regulations.

One of the most important interventions in maintaining sexual health is sex education, especially in addressing the increasing rates of HIV infection and other STDs among older adults. The best time to provide residents with sexual education materials is during the sexual history interview. The materials could include information about physiological changes related to aging that may affect the sexual experience as well as interventions that can maintain or restore sexual function (condoms, lubricants, medications). In addition, the materials should also provide information about how medications may interfere with sexual response and what steps can be taken to counter the effects. The person conducting the interview should also highlight the home's policies for honoring resident privacy.

HIV/AIDS AND OTHER SEXUALLY TRANSMITTED DISEASES

Before antiretroviral therapy was introduced to treat people with HIV, many lives were cut short, and people infected with the virus were not expected to live to old age. Because of this, older adults have seldom been seen as at risk for acquiring HIV/AIDS. More than 15% of the reported HIV/AIDS cases in the United States, however, are for individuals over the age of 50 (Kotz, 2007).

Despite the danger, older people continue to take risks with sexual activity. In a small study of unmarried women ages 58 to 93, nearly 60% said they had not used a condom the last time they had sex (Lindau, Leitsch, Lundberg, & Jerome, 2006). Another study showed that 27% of HIV-infected older men and 35% of HIV-infected older women sometimes have sex without using condoms (Lovejoy, 2007). Research following the sex lives of 624 older men between the ages of 49 and 80 found that 75% of them had had sexual activity with at least one partner in the previous 6 months (Cooperman, Arnsten, & Klein, 2007). Each of these men either had HIV or was at risk for acquiring it. Twenty-five percent of both HIV-positive and HIV-negative men had had more than one sexual partner. Only 18% of the HIV-negative men and 58% of the HIV-positive men used condoms every time they engaged in sexual intercourse. Other studies have shown that in older adults with at least one risk factor for HIV infection, only a small percentage use a condom during sexual activity or have undergone HIV testing (Mack & Ory, 2003; Stall & Catania, 1994).

Older people are less likely to know the risks for contracting the HIV/AIDS virus. The mortality rate for older adults with HIV/AIDS is very high, with 37% of patients over the age of 80 dying within 1 month of diagnosis (Zelenetz & Epstein, 1998). Older individuals who may be more likely to contract HIV share the following risk factors: (1) engage in unprotected sex; (2) share needles when doing illicit drugs; (3) received blood transfusions prior to 1986; (4) engage in male homosexual activity.

Older adults with HIV are more likely to be diagnosed later in the disease process, experience progression more quickly, and survive shorter periods of time than younger people (Zelenetz & Epstein, 1998). The delay in treating STDs in older adults may be the result of nurses and doctors not thinking to test for them and not expecting older adults to be at risk for developing them. For example, a male resident in a long-term care facility was treated for months for what nurses thought was a rash caused by incontinence. When treatments did not work, they finally diagnosed the problem as genital herpes. The delayed treatment may have caused further spread of the disease.

The following reasons have been cited for the increase in STDs in older adults (Resnick, 2003):

- Women past menopause cannot get pregnant and therefore choose not to use protection.

- The use of erectile dysfunction drugs has exploded since the late 1990s with the introduction of Viagra. The rate of STDs is twice as high in older men using these drugs as in their nonmedicated peers.

- There are more divorces and older people have better health, which have correlated with increased sexual activity.

- Today's seniors ignored the safe sex education of the 1980s as it related to the spread of HIV/AIDS and other STDs because they were settled in marriages and believed that STDs happened to other people.

- Older people were raised in a time when men made the decisions, and if men do not want to wear condoms, they do not have to.

- Women outnumber men, giving men far more options to choose from and to engage in sexual activity with. Women are sometimes willing to forego using protection to gain a competitive advantage over other women.

- Increasing numbers of older adults are finding partners via the Internet (Bodley-Tickell et al., 2008)

- Higher numbers of men are ignoring safe sex practices. Men in their 50s are six times more likely not to use condoms than men in their 20s. Rates of STDs have increased by 50% for men over age 50 since 1996 (Jena et al., 2010).

It is important to keep in mind that an STD may be present in an older adult even if he or she is not sexually active. For example, HIV may have been contracted through a blood transfusion. A resident may have tertiary syphilis and the initial infection may have occurred

> At least part of the blame for the increase in sexually transmitted diseases in older adults may be the reluctance on the part of the medical field to broach the subject of sexuality with older patients.

decades ago. And some STDs have no symptoms; a resident may not be aware that he or she is infected.

PREVENTION

Sex education materials for residents should also provide information on prevention. Residents can be taught that safe sex practices include sexual expression that does not involve an exchange of bodily fluids (e.g., massage, cuddling, mutual masturbation). Care staff can distribute material to residents on the proper use of a condom (Sidebars 9.2 and 9.3). Residents should also know that the best way to prevent the spread of STDs is through celibacy or a strictly monogamous relationship.

Sex therapist Kathryn Forsythe reports that older adults need to recognize that even condom use does not guarantee safe sex (personal communication, July 15, 2010). Because some older men lose their erections during sex, the condom can fall off during intercourse. These men need to be responsible for discontinuing intercourse to avoid an exchange of fluids. Orgasm can still be reached with masturbation and with the proper precautions.

Diagnosis is an essential part of a prevention strategy to reduce the risk of a resident passing an STD to another person. A resident's sexual history may alert staff to possible risks for infection. The Centers for Disease Control and Prevention released new HIV screening recommendations in September 2007, encouraging doctors to do voluntary blood tests for patients between the ages of 13 and 64 to prevent the spread of new infections by those who are unaware they have the virus (see For Further Information at the back of the book). Long-term care facilities can offer voluntary HIV screening for residents. Screening can also be offered for other STDs. If an STD is diagnosed, treatment and counseling can be offered to a resident. Care staff should encourage residents to alert them to the presence of any rash, sore, blister, or discharge. It is also important to seek out, evaluate, treat, and counsel any sexual partners of a resident who is diagnosed with an STD.

DISCUSSION

Can you think of an intervention that could have prevented Charlie from refusing to take his blood pressure medication in an effort to maintain his sexual performance? What type of sex education do you think is important for the residents you now serve and for the baby boomers who are beginning to arrive to your facility?

SUMMARY

Skeptics of the need to provide sex education to residents living in long-term care will have the most difficulty with this chapter. Many residents themselves will not

Sidebar 9.2
Recommendations from the Centers for Disease Control and Prevention for the Use of Condoms

1. Only latex condoms should be used. "Natural skin" condoms have pores that are large enough for HIV and other infections to pass through.
2. Condoms must be used during vaginal, oral, or rectal sex.
3. Condoms should contain, or be used in conjunction with, 5% nonoxynol 9, which has been shown to kill HIV and other infectious diseases.
4. The expiration date should be checked. Do not use outdated condoms.
5. Store condoms in a cool, dry place.
6. Have condoms available at all times and discard after each use.
7. The condom should be placed on an erect penis. As the condom is rolled onto the penis, the tip of the condom should be held to squeeze out the air, leaving space for the ejaculate. The entire penis, to the hair, must be covered.
8. Only water-soluble lubricants, such as K-Y Jelly or nonoxynol-9, should be used. Oil-based lubricants, such as Vaseline, cause disintegration of the condom.
9. After ejaculation, the condom should be removed while the penis is still erect.
10. Unlubricated condoms should be used during oral sex. Nonoxynol-9 may be placed inside the condom before oral sex but should not be on the outside.

Source: U.S. Department of Health and Human Services, Public Health Services. (1988). Condoms for the prevention of sexually transmitted diseases. *Morbidity and Mortality Weekly Report, 37*(9), 133–137.

see a need and may think the administration is out of line in addressing the subject of sexual health and safe sex practices. There are some residents, however, who will be interested in ways to maintain their sexual health; they will be happy that their facility is following a whole-person care philosophy.

Activity and education staff can develop activities to encourage a deeper commitment to and understanding of sexual health and wellness among residents,

Sidebar 9.3
Condom Use

Some persons may have trouble reading or understanding the instructions for condom use and may need verbal instructions from a nurse or physician. Use the Centers for Disease Control and Prevention recommendations to learn the proper way to place a condom using a banana.

The following recommendations for safe sex may be included with any sex education program or materials provided by a long-term care facility:

RECOMMENDATIONS FOR SAFE SEX

- Know your partner.
- Limit the number of sexual partners.
- Avoid the exchange of body fluids.
- Use condoms and spermicidal ointment or foam for all sexual activity.
- Practice good hygiene; wash the genital area before and after sex.
- See your physician yearly for medical checkups.

Source: Letvak, S., & Schoder, D. (1996). Sexually transmitted diseases in the elderly: What you need to know. *Geriatric Nursing, 17*(4), 156–160. Reprinted with permission.

as well as to launch sex education programming. For example, residents can be introduced to Strip Bingo. The game is played by stripping the called out items from a board until one player has stripped an entire row. A wet T-shirt contest, as described at the beginning of the chapter, might also garner some attention.

REFERENCES

Bodley-Tickell, A., Olowokure, B., Bhaduri, S., White, D., Ward, D., Ross, J. et al. (2008). Trends in sexually transmitted infections (other than HIV) in older people: Analysis of data from an enhanced surveillance system. *Sexually Transmitted Infections, 84,* 312–317.

Cooperman, N., Arnsten, J., & Klein, R. (2007). Current sexual activity and risky sexual behavior in older men with or at risk for HIV infection. *AIDS Education Preview, 19*(4), 321–333.

Delamater, J., & Moorman, S. (2007). Sexual behavior in later life. *Journal of Aging and Health, 19,* 921–945.

Haleem, S. (2004). Urinary incontinence in older adults: Prevalence, severity, quality of life issues, and treatment seeking behavior among Medicare beneficiaries. *Public Health and the Environment.* Retrieved from http://apha.confex.com/apha/132am/techprogram/paper_79049.htm.

Jena, A., Goldman, D., Kamdar, A., Lakdawalla, D., & Lu, Y. (2010). Sexually transmitted diseases among users of erectile dysfunction drugs: Analysis of claims data. *Annals of Internal Medicine, 153,* 1–7.

Kotz, D. (2007). Sex ed for seniors: You still need those condoms; Sexually transmitted diseases stalk older singles, too. *U.S. News and World Report, 143*(5), 45.

Letvak, S., & Schoder, D. (1996). Sexually transmitted diseases in the elderly: What you need to know. *Geriatric Nursing, 17*(4), 156–160.

Lindau, S., Leitsch, S., Lundberg, K., & Jerome, J. (2006). Older women's attitudes, behavior, and communication about sex and HIV: A community-based study. *Journal of Women's Health, 15*(6), 747–753.

Lovejoy, T. (2007). Patterns and correlates of sexual activity and condom use behavior in persons 50-plus years of age living with HIV/AIDS. Retrieved from http://etd.ohiolink.edu/view.cgi?acc_num=ohiou1193840743.

Mack, K., & Ory, M. (2003). AIDS and older Americans at the end of the twentieth century. *Journal of Acquired Immune Deficiency Syndromes, 33*(suppl. 2), S68–75.

Resnick, B. (2003). Risky behaviors in older adults. Medscape. Retrieved from http://cme.medscape.com/viewarticle/464727.

Stall, R., & Catania, J. (1994). AIDS risk behaviors among late middle-aged and elderly Americans: The national AIDS behavioral surveys. *Archives of Internal Medicine, 154*(1), 57–63.

U.S. Department of Health and Human Services, Public Health Services. (1988). Condoms for the prevention of sexually transmitted diseases. *MMWR Morbidity and Mortality Weekly Report, 37*(9), 133–137.

Wallace, M. A. (2008). Assessment of sexual health in older adults: Using the PLISSIT model to talk about sex. *American Journal of Nursing, 108*(7), 52–60.

Zelenetz, P., & Epstein, M. (1998). HIV in the elderly. *AIDS Patient Care STDS. 12*(4), 255–262.

What's Normal? Card Game

It has been said that 30% of aging is genetic and 70% comes from the lifestyle a person lives. This game helps residents and staff members to understand what types of changes associated with aging are normal and which are pathological or due to a disease process. This activity identifies all types of changes, not just those associated with sexuality, because a game focused solely on sex may be too uncomfortable for some participants.

For the game you will need to purchase two decks of cards and some light-colored contact paper. Cover the numbered side of all the cards with contact paper. (The best way to do this is to lay the contact paper on a counter sticky-side up and place the cards down on the paper. Then trim around the edges of the card.) Using a marker pen, write one of the conditions or aging changes from the following lists on each card.

Normal Aging	Pathological Aging
Wrinkles	Diabetes
Age spots	Constipation
Increased reaction time	Cataracts
Loss of vaginal elasticity and lubrication	Significant hearing loss
White or gray hair	Arthritis
Presbyopia	Prostate cancer
Slowed sexual response	Glaucoma

Decrease in penile sensitivity

Liver spots

Decrease in sexual desire

Lower basal metabolic rate (BMI)

Delayed erections

Breast cancer

Heart disease

Hypertension

Gout

Alzheimer's disease

Stroke

Dementia

Depression

Significant sensory losses

Cancer

Impotence

Under Normal Aging are changes that happen to all of us as we get older. The conditions listed under Pathological Aging are a result of disease. Although they tend to develop more frequently with age, they are not caused by age.

Shuffle the cards together and do not reveal to participants which cards are from the Normal Aging pile and which are from Pathological Aging. Deal five cards, written side down, to each person. Say to the participants, "These are the cards you've been dealt in your life." Have them review the cards and exchange those that are obviously for the opposite gender for another card from the deck (i.e., if a female participant has a card for prostate cancer).

Next, ask the participants to lay down any cards with conditions that they think are examples of pathological aging. Explain what pathological aging is and answer any questions participants may have about conditions they do not understand. Ask participants to share which cards they have left; they should all be conditions from the Normal Aging list. Discuss which changes or conditions normally occur with aging and what can be done about each. At the end of the game you will have provided some sex education without too much shock value, which may open the door to further education in the future.

Sexuality and Long-Term Care: Understanding and Supporting the Needs of Older Adults, by Gayle Appel Doll
(Copyright 2012, by Health Professions Press, Inc.)

10

Policy

OBJECTIVES

- Define the steps needed to develop a sexuality policy for a long-term care organization
- Determine the people who need to be engaged in the process of policy development
- Discuss how to draft a policy
- Review sample policies

*A*dministrator Janice was at the breaking point. For months she had been dealing with a resident issue that seemed to get more out of hand with each passing day. A family member had taken a complaint to the nursing home's ombudsman, who had been unable to resolve the matter. It now seemed as though the whole state was involved.

It all began when Alice was found in a compromising position with Clarence in his room. Before Janice had a chance to provide a calming influence, a staff member had reported the behavior to Alice's family, and they were insisting that Clarence be moved from the home. Alice had been a very proper woman who had been devoted to her church prior to her admission to the home. Her family felt certain that Clarence had taken advantage of her decreased cognitive state.

Staff members were divided about the problem. Some agreed that Clarence should leave or at least be moved to an area in the building where he and Alice were not likely to meet. Others were not so sure. They felt that Alice was still capable of making some decisions and that her relationship with Clarence was not hurting anyone; in fact, it seemed to be very beneficial to her and Clarence's well-being.

The ombudsman appeared to know very little about older adult sexuality but tried to do the best she could to get the family to consider both sides of the issue. This they *refused to do. In the meantime, Clarence's family refused to budge as well, insisting that Clarence had never demonstrated this type of behavior prior to Alice moving in, which meant it was likely Alice who was the instigator.*

 Poor Janice felt torn between her loyalty to the two residents, who clearly seemed happy with each other, and to their families, who were desperately trying to hang onto the parents they had known and loved. She couldn't help but wonder if she and the staff would have been better prepared to address the issue if the facility had a resident sexuality policy.

WHY IS POLICY IMPORTANT?

The desire to concede to a resident's wishes, especially if it makes the person happy, is natural and understandable. It would be nice if that could simply be the policy, but such a policy would fail to address potential harm or offense to a resident or staff member. In an institutional environment harm or offense can come in many forms. There could be harm to a resident who expresses him- or herself sexually. There is also potential harm or offense to a resident who may be the object of another resident's desire, as well as to others in the home (residents, staff) or to family members or friends of a resident. Potential harm to the self has been the area most frequently examined by long-term care organizations, specifically a resident's ability to consent. Most policies not only assess for ability to consent, but also the residents' ability to understand the potential risks in having an intimate relationship. Many policies, however, do not take into consideration potential harm or offense to others.

> Long-term care organizations are pledged to protect residents from harm as well as to ensure that residents' rights of autonomy and self-determination are honored. From a legal perspective, then, sexual expression policies must respect residents' sexual needs, and at the same time protect them from harm.

 Harm or offense to residents may result from an abusive relationship. For staff members it may result from taking offense at being instructed to support a relationship they think is morally wrong (see Chapter 7, Lesbian, Gay, Bisexual, and Transgendered Residents). Advocates for nursing home residents have suggested that interference in these matters should occur only if there is significant harm or offense to others and if the harm is greater than the benefits of allowing a resident to do what he or she wants.

 Jane and Paul started "going together," which was OK with everyone, including their families, as long as they kept separate residences in their as-

sisted living home. When they both began to decline cognitively at the same time and became candidates for dementia care, the administrator suggested they live together to save money. Jane's family agreed, but Paul's son said no; he was worried about how they would be perceived by others in the community. At no point were Jane and Paul asked about what they wanted.

The decision to discourage, promote, or ignore a sexual relationship is often made between the resident's family and the long-term care home's administration and staff, and is frequently independent of the resident's choice.

Sometimes it appears as though long-term care facilities make decisions based on the wishes of family members and not those of the resident. If a family member directs a home to put an end to a loved one's behavior, administrators and staff work to make it happen. If family members are supportive of a loved one's relationship with another resident in the home, the facility respects and is supportive of the relationship as well. The belief has primarily been that adult children of residents are the primary consumers of long-term care, and so they need to be catered to. Long-term care facilities, however, have increasingly been forced to abandon this approach to accommodate the needs of the growing aging population and its demands for appropriate housing and care environments.

An intentional and well-conceived sexuality policy ensures that the proper steps will be taken to meet residents' needs. The process for addressing resident sexuality should also take into consideration the needs and values of staff and family members. Thus, the knee-jerk reactions that sometimes occur in response to resident sexual behavior can be reduced. In addition, a written policy can clearly state the organization's commitment to meeting the needs of the whole person. Perhaps no other policy can convey this message as strongly. It may even attract potential new residents to the home. Older adults may feel more comfortable moving to a long-term care facility that recognizes and supports their sexuality (Sidebar 10.1).

STEPS INVOLVED IN DEVELOPING A SEXUALITY POLICY

A long-term care organization's current practice may not lead to the best outcomes for residents. Policy development can help in considering all sides of an issue related

Sidebar 10.1
Kansas State University Center on Aging Research

In the Center on Aging research project at Kansas State University, nursing home administrators and staff were asked if the home they worked for had a sexuality policy. We were surprised when 26% responded yes. When we asked what the policy was, it appeared that very few of the homes had in fact developed specific policies to address resident sexuality. Most of those surveyed were using resident rights policies. Responses were as follows:

- Resident rights
- Firstly, mutual consent must be present. We are to provide privacy to the best of our ability and we will perform any assistance within the scope of our regular duties.
- Allow conjugal visits
- Allow free sexual expression between residents with the mental ability to reasonably consent
- The residents have the right to practice what their sexual orientation is. They have the right to privacy and confidentiality. As a facility we are to be supportive and honor our residents' wishes.
- Procedures are as follows per policy
- Privacy and consensual, family notification if dementia is present
- Related to married couples only because we are a Christian and church-related facility
- It is not specific but it states that if a person wishes to be sexually active it is fine as long as all parties involved give consent.
- Right of choice and privacy
- Partners may share rooms if they both agree. We will not discriminate by race, creed, or sexual orientation. Residents have the right to privacy.

It is clear from this list that nursing home staff in Kansas have very little specific written guidance when it comes to resident sexual expression.

to resident sexuality. The first step in creating a policy is to assemble a team of the key stakeholders. Volunteers can be assembled from the following list:

Health care or personal support worker	Family
Nutritionist or dietician	Administrator
Housekeeper	Board representative
Registered nurse	Pastoral care representative
Licensed practical nurse	Volunteer coordinator
Social worker	Ethicist
Recreational therapist	Residents
Physiotherapist	Ombudsmen
Physician	

It is interesting to note that when Center on Aging staff asked Kansas nursing home administrators who was responsible for creating what few policies we were able to find as part of our research, no one had included residents or ombudsmen in the creation of the standards (Activity 10.1).

The next step in policy development is to learn as much as possible about older adult sexuality. It will be important to confront personal biases and pre-existing beliefs about sexuality and aging. This book should be beneficial for conducting such a review and for initiating discussions. It may also be helpful to have a professional facilitator to guide discussions that will arise during policy development.

It may be the ultimate paternalistic insult that long-term care organizations create rules and policies governing resident sexuality without permitting residents to participate in the process. The organization should develop a plan for resident input, whether it be through surveys, interviews, focus groups, or representation on the policy-writing team.

The policy development team may conduct focus group meetings to encourage other staff members to discuss their values, beliefs, and personal moral codes. Issues of consent and risk assessment could also be discussed in these sessions. This step assesses the "culture" of the home and helps to determine what administrators and staff deem as normal and acceptable behaviors as well as inappropriate or pathological behaviors.

One of the goals for the focus groups may be to examine existing policies that impede intimacy in the long-term care environment. For example, some facilities follow a medical model and offer only single beds for more efficient caregiving, which is definitely a barrier to sexual activity.

Following these discussions the group should review sexuality policies from other organizations. For example, the Hebrew Home at Riverdale in the Bronx, New York, formalized their resident rights to sexual expression in 1995 (Sidebar 10.2). Nearly every other effort on the part of other long-term care organizations to protect and support resident sexuality has arisen from the home's advocacy efforts. Each organization's policies will include features that are specific to its own unique characteristics. It may also be helpful to view policies that have been developed for other population segments, such as people with developmental disabilities. The disabilities movement has stressed the right to control all aspects of one's life, including sexual expression.

Policies should be developed and modified over time with future populations in mind. Baby boomers and other coming generations, for example, may request less protective policies and practices regarding their sexuality in return for greater autonomy and control. Given the differing characteristics of the cohort currently using long-term care and those of the baby boom generation who have begun to enter it, special attention may need to be paid to honoring individual needs.

Policies will also differ based on level of care. The sexuality policies for an assisted living facility certainly would look different from those of a skilled nursing facility. For example, assisted living generally has minimal policies regarding sexuality, and they are usually informal. In current practice assisted living directors instruct their staffs to leave quietly when they observe sexual behavior in residents' apartments. They are, however, expected to report this activity to supervisors. The reason given is that if something were to happen, they would have documentation about it. Family members are also informed as a matter of course, and frequently care planning meetings are set up (sometimes without the resident present). In some cases, families will give permission for their loved one to engage in sex.

A particularly difficult task in the development of policy is determining working definitions of key concepts to be included in the policy. It will be important for the team to determine the differences between sexuality, intimacy, and sexual behavior, and to decide which behaviors are normal and acceptable and which are not. The group will also have to outline how to determine consent for sexual activity (Sidebar 10.3). (Guidelines for this can be found in Chapter 5.)

Identifying the appropriate staff interventions or responses to sexual behavior is the next step in the policy development process. This may require listing each type of sexual expression and determining the appropriate response for each. For example, what should staff do when they find two women holding hands, or two cognitively intact residents engaged in oral sex (Activity 10.2)?

Sidebar 10.2
The Hebrew Home at Riverdale

The Hebrew Home at Riverdale in the Bronx, New York, created a team of diverse positions and expertise to establish policies and procedures to address resident sexuality. The team included social workers, psychiatric nurses, therapeutic recreation specialists, researchers, residents' families, and religious representatives. They first interviewed staff and then assigned the following tasks to different team members:

- Create a formal policy that gives rights to residents for sexual expression with caveats regarding cognitive impairments.

- Develop a staff education program intended to help staff be more responsive to resident sexual needs.

- Modify the physical environment to facilitate resident sexuality and intimacy.

- Implement family orientation to explain the needs and rights of older adults to sexual expression and intimacy.

The team then formed an interdisciplinary work group that met over a 7-month period to review literature and develop a questionnaire that was used to gauge attitudes about resident sexuality. They then worked together to develop a resident sexuality policy. The primary challenge they faced was to create a policy that was general yet clear, had the ability to show support without seeming to give license, and limited boundaries while being inclusive.

The group developed the following definition for *sexual expression*: "words, gestures or movements (including reaching, pursuing, or touching) which appear motivated by the desire for sexual gratification."

Key elements of the policy they created are as follows:

- Residents have a right to privacy and to sexual and intimate relationships (for all sexual orientations).

- Staff and the facility have specific responsibilities.

(continued on next page)

Sidebar 10.2 (continued)

- Sexual expression may be between or among residents or may include visitors from outside the home.

- Residents have a right to access and/or obtain for private use materials with legal but sexually explicit content: magazines, films, videos, pictures, or drawings.

- To the greatest extent possible, residents have the right to access facilities, most notably private space, in support of sexual expression.

Creating an environment for residents to express their sexuality reflects the home's commitment to the happiness and quality of life of its residents, a fundamental pillar of the person-centered care approach. Hebrew Home at Riverdale was commissioned to develop a training video titled *Freedom of Sexual Expression: Dementia and Resident Rights in Long-Term Facilities* (see For Further Information at the back of the book).

Writing the Policy

When all the information has been gathered the work group can begin to draft a working policy document. A good place to start is by ensuring that a specific reference to sexual expression is written into the organization's mission statement. There are also certain situations that should be addressed by the organizational policy, including the following:

Admissions.   During admissions is the best time to gather information about new residents, including sexual orientation, sleeping arrangements at home, and current level of sexual interest and activity. Family members and residents should be assured that this information is necessary to make a successful transition to the home. This process will not go over well if the home has not been very open about the fact that they have a sexuality policy that includes asking questions about residents' sexual history to better protect and support residents' needs. The policy should be clearly stated in organization brochures and literature as well as posted to the organization's website. For a truly person-centered approach, however, these questions should be regarded as optional. Each resident has the right to privacy regarding their sexual history.

Sidebar 10.3
New Possibilities

The group developing a home's sexuality policy will need to define how the ability to consent should be determined and by whom. Frequently consent ability is measured using the Mini-Mental State Examination (MMSE) (see Chapter 5). Some ethicists claim that the overreliance on tests of cognitive ability dehumanizes and discriminates against those with dementia. The quality of connections to others may be a better indicator of cognitive functioning and consent ability. People with dementia may still be functional in relationships due to semantic memory, where people assign meaning to what they experience in the present, unrelated to past history. Residents with dementia may also exhibit behaviors that are inconsistent with their age group or with their behavior prior to the onset of the disease. But while these new behaviors and ways of connecting with others may be unsettling to family and friends, they could instead be understood as new possibilities rather than just pathology, which may ease the isolation and loss of dementia by continuing to allow people with the disease to experience closeness and intimacy.

Consent.   Chapter 5 discusses some of the methods for determining consent. Staff members will want to explore these strategies and make a decision about the course of action that is best suited to their organization and the needs of the resident. It is important to recognize that some of the methods require a resident to have the ability to articulate his or her needs (e.g., the Lichtenberg decision tree). In the early 1990s, a national nursing home chain convened a task force to develop staff guidelines for its dementia special care units to assess residents' ability to consent. They developed four key principles:

1. Sexual expression should be allowed if both parties and their family members consent and if the benefits outweigh the risks.

2. Care staff may decide whether to permit sexual behavior or activity and should draw upon family guidance.

3. Staff members will be responsible for determining and documenting consent, for discussing risks with the resident and family members, and for developing a care plan.

4. The organization will work to find a mutually agreeable solution when family members object to consensual behavior between residents.

Risk.   There should be an assessment procedure to determine the level of risk associated with sexual behavior. The policy may include a determination of what level of risk is acceptable or it can more broadly state that the risk level would be determined on an individual basis.

Shared rooms.   The policy may include stipulations to address a resident's desire to share a room with someone he or she is engaged in an intimate relationship with. There may be additional policies for conjugal visit rooms.

Staff training.   The organization policy should address the type and frequency of training required of staff regarding resident sexuality. Because of high turnover in the long-term care industry, it is important for staff training to be repeated. The policy may also include expectations for staff participation.

Reporting procedure.   How will reports of observed sexual behavior be handled? When will families be informed? What documentation procedures will be used? It may be necessary to stipulate the appropriate terminology to use when recording observations and how to avoid personal bias in written statements. The documentation system should detail frequency, intensity, duration, and level of risk associated with the observed sexual behavior.

Sexual ethics committee.   An organization may choose to call this group by some other name, but it is important that a team be assembled to review instances of sexual expression and to identify, implement, and evaluate possible interventions, as required. It is important to include family or substitute decision makers as well as the resident in these discussion groups (Activity 10.3).

Police involvement.   The policy should include the types of circumstances related to sexual behavior that might warrant calling the police or other investigative body.

Resident sexual education and support.   As discussed in Chapter 9, residents who choose to engage in sexual activity should be taught the risks of spreading sexually transmitted diseases. Many are unaware of the risks and will need to learn safe sex practices. Resident sex education should also include information about the physiological changes that are a normal part of aging and how they may affect sexual performance, as well as the affects of certain medications on sexual function.

Case studies. It is a good idea to include case studies as an addendum to the policy. They can be used in staff training and orientation.

Sidebars 10.4 and 10.5 at the end of the chapter are examples of sexuality policies from different long-term care organizations that key stakeholders can review and use in developing policy.

Implementing Policy

Once the draft of the policy is completed, the work group should circulate it to staff, the resident council, and family members for their input. Take the time to gather feedback and revisit and modify the drafted policy. It might be useful to invite a speaker to address the administration and staff as a kick-off once the final version of the policy is complete. An organization could also sponsor an annual sexual awareness event, during which the policy and other sexuality training could be reviewed.

It will be difficult to please everyone with any set of policies but it does not mean that an organization should ignore the need for them. "If residents merely live in the *staff's place of employment*, then such personal matters can be disregarded. Alternatively, if staff members work in the *resident's home*, every consideration will be given to understanding and meeting their needs. A facility's basic philosophy on this central issue can help define whether care facilities are primarily public or private places and determine how policies and guidelines are formulated and enacted."
(Kuhn, 2002, p. 168)

Evaluation of Policy and Practice

Good policies are always works in progress. The work group should arrange to have a feedback mechanism that will assist in revising the policy over time (Activity 10.4). The policy should be reviewed at least every 2 years to see if it adequately reflects the current understanding of sexual expression in long-term care.

Ballard (1996) listed the following indicators for whether a care facility has adopted a respectful approach to resident sexuality:

- The organization enhances resident well-being using a holistic approach that considers the social, emotional, spiritual, physical, and sexual needs.

- Staff members feel comfortable addressing resident needs for intimacy and sexuality and can use strategies for dealing with specific situations that involve residents and their families.

- The organization's administration has established guidelines for policies and practices for resolving dilemmas involving intimate relationships between residents.

- Families and legal guardians have a clear understanding prior to a resident's admission of the potential for intimate relationships and the organization's policies on such matters. A sexual history profile is completed on admission.

SUMMARY

Developing a sexuality policy and related staff training are essential to understanding and supporting the needs of residents. Both require hard work and persistence, and the work is not done when the policy has been created and the training has been implemented. The policy and training will need to be reevaluated regularly over time to ensure they retain their effectiveness. The ultimate result will be residents and families who are satisfied with the care the home provides.

REFERENCES

Ballard, E. L. (1996). Sexuality in the special care unit. In: S. B. Hoffman & M. Kaplan, (Eds.). *Special care programs for people with dementia* (pp. 255–270). Baltimore: Health Professions Press.

Frankowski, A. C., & Clark, L. (2009). Sexuality and intimacy in assisted living; Residents' perspectives and experiences. *Sexuality Research and Social Policy,* 6(4), 25–37.

Hebrew Home at Riverdale (1995). Policies and procedures concerning sexual expression at the Hebrew Home for the Aged at Riverdale. Retrieved from www.agingkansas.org/.../ PEAK/Modules/sexualitymodulef.pdf

Ingersoll, T., & Scott, S. (n.d.) Sexuality policy guidelines for a geriatric residential facility. Retrieved from http://www.scribd.com/doc/18551910/Sample-Geriatric-Residence-Sexuality-Policy

Kuhn, F. (2002, spring). Intimacy, sexuality, and residents with dementia. *Alzheimer's Care Quarterly,* 3(2) 165–173.

Sidebar 10.4

Sample Sexuality Policy for a Geriatric Residential Facility

- Residents have the right to seek out and engage in sexual expression, including physical affection, emotional intimacy, sexual intercourse, and masturbation. They have the right to develop relationships and make decisions pertaining to the nature of those relationships. Their sexuality shall not be limited by the parameters of heteronormativity, and should include alternative orientation and identity expressions such as gay, lesbian, bisexual, transgender, queer, and intersex.

- Residents have the right to live in environments that facilitate physical and emotional privacy in the area of human relations and sexuality. This could simply be in the form of having "do not disturb" signs hung onto room doors, which would need to be respected by staff. Another option would be to allow conjugal visits within the residence, or through visitations outside the residence. When possible, providing residents with private rooms with larger beds may offer a solution. In addition, there is the option of having spare rooms set aside for the privacy of the residents.

- Residents have the right to engage in sexual activity without fear of punishment and/or public ridicule by residential staff. Sexual expression may occur individually (i.e., masturbation), between or among residents, or may include visitors. Encouragement for other forms of sexual expression, such as hugging or kissing, should be permitted. However, sexual acts that include minors, those that are not consensual, and sexual activity between people who are cognitively impaired to the point of being deemed unable to give consent are not allowed. Furthermore, sexual expressions that negatively impact the residential community as a whole, such as through public display, are prohibited. Any sexual contact between staff and residents is also unacceptable and will be dealt with immediately and severely upon discovery.

(continued on next page)

Sidebar 10.4 (continued)

- Residents have the right to access and/or obtain sexually explicit material for private use, as long as they are considered legal by the states in which they are purchased. Such material may include books, magazines, film, video, pictures, or drawings. Residents also have the right to sexual education by qualified and competent educators, or by staff trained by such educators, who can answer residents' questions about topics such as sexuality, sexual function, medication sexual side effects, sexually transmitted infections (STI), contraception/STI prevention barrier methods, alternative sexual lifestyles, sexual orientation, gender, sexual anatomy and self-pleasuring.

Source: Ingersoll, T. S., & Scott, S. (2009). Sexuality policy guidelines for a geriatric residential facility. Retrieved from http://www.scribd.com/doc/18551910/Sample-Geriatric-Residence-Sexuality-Policy. Reprinted with permission. (http://www.travisskyingersoll.com)

Sample Sexuality Policy

(Name of Facility and Date)

POLICY MEMORANDUM

Intimate Relationships of and Sexual Activities by Residents

Purpose
To affirm the facility's support for the intimate relationships of and sexual activities by the residents.

Policies
1. The facility supports and places no unreasonable conditions on the sexual activities of the residents.

2. The facility provides both anticipatory and situational supports for the intimate relationships and sexual activities of the residents.

3. The facility provides appropriate risk-related heath information to residents and their healthcare surrogates relating to its residents' intimate relationships and sexual activities.

4. The facility provides staff training and education regarding this policy, the procedure and the role of staff in relationship to this policy, and related procedures.

5. Notwithstanding its policy of providing support for its residents' sexual activities, some resident sexual activities may be so problematic that they cannot be supported.

6. Upon admission, the facility informs the resident's primary contact person of policies 1 and 2.

7. Upon admission, the facility seeks information from the resident's primary contact person that may be helpful in anticipating and supporting the resident's intimate relationships and sexual activities.

8. The facility informs the primary contact person of observed sexual contact involving the resident.

(continued on next page)

Sidebar 10.5 *(continued)*

9. The facility's care-plan process includes review of the intimate relationships and sexual activities of residents.

10. The facility's policies concerning abuse, including sexual abuse, are contained in separate policy memoranda.

11. The facility will assess whether observed intimate relationships or sexual activities are abusive. Each such assessment will be documented.

Source: Center for Practical Bioethics. (2006). Considerations regarding the needs of long-term care residents for intimate relationships and sexual activity. Retrieved from http://www.practicalabioethics. org/wp-content/uploads/2011/07/Intimacy_Guidelines_Aug2007.pdf. Reprinted with permission.

Stakeholders

Working in a group, make a list of people you think should be involved in writing a resident sexuality policy and the role each could contribute. Keep in mind that the larger the team, the more difficult it will be to manage and the more time it will take to reach consensus. If you have a large group, you may want to break it up into work or action groups. One group might be assigned to do the background work, collecting information about pre-existing policies and perhaps conducting focus groups within the facility. Another group might be tasked with doing the actual writing.

Sexuality and Long-Term Care: Understanding and Supporting the Needs of Older Adults, by Gayle Appel Doll
(Copyright 2012, by Health Professions Press, Inc.)

Interventions

List the types of sexual expression that frequently occur in your long-term care setting. In a small group discuss the appropriate interventions for each. It is acceptable to write "no intervention required." Add other potential behaviors to the list as well.

SEXUAL EXPRESSION   **INTERVENTION**

Handholding, heterosexual _____

_____

_____

_____

Handholding, homosexual _____

_____

_____

_____

Masturbating, public _____

_____

_____

_____

Masturbating, private _____

_____

_____

_____

Oral sex, two consenting residents _____

_____

_____

_____

Oral sex, one resident with dementia _____

_____

_____

_____

Others _____

_____

_____

_____

Ethics Committee Discussion

In a small group develop a protocol for discussing types of sexual expression that have caused concern in your long-term care setting. The discussion should include descriptions of observed behaviors from people on the team, including from family members, as well as an assessment of the competency of the residents involved. The team may want to review the beliefs and values of the resident, family, and staff to identify any differences in how the behaviors are perceived and how these differences might affect the committee's decision-making process. What do participants think should happen in this situation? An important question to ask may be, "Given the differences, what are the circumstances under which the relationship or behaviors could be allowed to continue?" Finally, the participants will identify, implement, and evaluate possible interventions to address specific situations and describe what the acceptable outcomes would be for each intervention.

Sexuality and Long-Term Care: Understanding and Supporting the Needs of Older Adults, by Gayle Appel Doll (Copyright 2012, by Health Professions Press, Inc.)

Your Turn

Take any of the case stories that begin the chapters of this book and discuss how having a sexuality policy in place can improve an organization's ability to make clear decisions in supporting the needs of residents. After the group has become convinced of the importance of such policies, begin the process of developing policy for your organization using the steps outlined in this chapter.

Final Thoughts

Max and Harriet had been married for more than 40 years when they began to realize that her forgetfulness might actually be Alzheimer's disease. Harriet decides that she must go to a nursing home after she gets lost and realizes that she is at risk. The assisted living facility that she chooses has a no-visitation policy for the first 30 days so that a new resident can adjust to his or her new situation. Max is not happy about the policy but accepts the condition to appease his wife. When he returns to visit her 30 days later she seemingly has forgotten him and has become attached to Clarence, another man in the home. Max suspects that she is doing this purposely so that she can punish him for his past infidelities. He continues to visit but feels like a voyeur in her new life. When Clarence's wife moves him out of the facility for financial reasons, Harriet goes into a deep depression. Max, wanting to make his wife happy, meets with Clarence and his wife at their home and asks her to allow Clarence to visit Harriet.

Does this story sound familiar? It is the plot for the 2006 movie *Away from Her*. It was released at about the same time Justice Sandra Day O'Conner announced that her husband of 45 years had Alzheimer's disease and had fallen in love with a woman living in his assisted living facility. Justice O'Conner expressed her support for the relationship because it made her husband happy.

These two events seemed to herald a new interest in sexuality in long-term care. In a review of the literature, this does not appear to be the first time for this fascination. A sizable body of research dates to the 1990s, but a lapse occurred for about a decade, with renewed interest after 2005. It is hard to say why the earlier interest failed to take root and lead to policy and education for key stakeholders in long-term care.

Times are changing, and from a personal perspective I can sense the change. From the time I began to investigate sexuality and aging in 2008, there has been a tremendous interest in information related to older adult sexuality. I have been called an expert in the field largely, I believe, because so few others have explored this topic. I was asked to join a consortium on sexuality and aging, and have been invited to lecture at conferences. It seems as though every participant at these presentations has a story to tell. People appear to be ready to bring sexuality and aging "out of the closet."

Much of the interest on the part of people working in long-term care has come about because there has been so little guidance for how to respond when sexual expression becomes a problem. Nearly all professional caregivers have chosen long-term care because of a desire to help people. Most of the rules about how to provide that care are standard and easy to understand. For the most part, however, sexual expression has not been considered a part of the care environment. There are no rules, no training, and no orientation to guide and direct caregiver behaviors and interventions that are person centered.

Sexuality in long-term care has been consistent over time. There has always been a need for intimacy and sexuality in older residents, and there have always been residents who have acted on those needs. And such will continue to be the case, but the support and understanding from administrators and staff to fulfill those needs currently is limited, if they exist at all.

The changes that are now occurring appear to be in the attitudes of caregivers, who are beginning to recognize that sexual intimacy is normal and benefits residents. The alignment of this renewed interest with the current culture change movement that emphasizes person-centered care may be the impetus for sustained efforts to understand sexuality as a basic human need of older residents (Sidebar 11.1). Failing to consider sexuality as a critical factor in the lives of older adults is a product of socialization.

As I was wrapping up this final chapter, I received a phone call from a newspaper reporter. He was writing an article about a 100-year-old woman who was going about her life as if she were 20 years younger. He wanted my opinion on

Sidebar 11.1
Our Ah-Ha Moment

The Kansas State University Center on Aging has been producing training materials for long-term care since 2000. These materials are focused on person-centered care. The movement to this model of care has been called *culture change.* We started the training process by giving a broad overview of what culture change is, and then we went to more specific aspects of how to provide care and honor resident needs. It is perhaps symbolic of the lack of societal recognition of older adult sexuality that we had written 10 training modules, ranging from staffing practices to environments to spirituality, before it occurred to us that we needed to address this important aspect of human behavior.

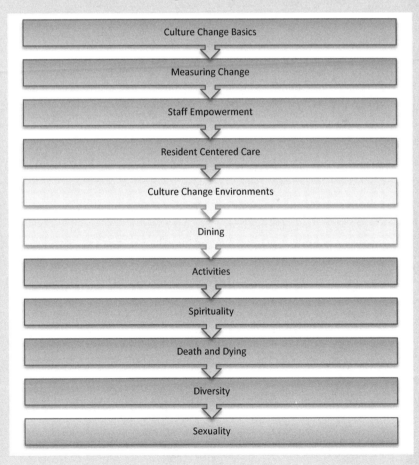

how it was that she was able to do that. I told him the standard things about genetic predisposition and healthy lifestyles, but I also told him that I think chronological age is losing its significance, except for bragging rights. What matters perhaps the most is one's social age. We are socialized by our families, peers, the media, and our own predispositions to believe that certain behaviors are appropriate at certain ages. We are told repeatedly in myriad ways to "act your age."

The 100-year-old woman clearly was not listening whenever anyone told her she should be "resting" or "retiring to a quiet life." And she was not listening when her doctors told her "after all, you're not getting any younger." She just chose to live her life and on her own terms.

I believe we are on the cusp of a cultural revolution regarding older adult sexuality. We are told that 60 is the new 40. We look at ourselves and see people who are far younger than our parents were at our age (socially and physically). We are living our lives outside the cultural norms of what is or is not appropriate for the number of years we have lived. More and more older people will recognize that they can enjoy a sexual life long beyond the time at which society has told them they should no longer be interested.

And that is why this book. We need to be ready.

For Further Information

Chapter 1. Introduction

American Psychological Association. Aging and human sexuality resource guide. This guide lists articles, books, book chapters, organizations, and other resources. (http://www.apa.org/pi/aging/resources/guides/sexuality.aspx)

Consortium for Sexuality and Aging at Widener University. This consortium seeks to provide education for older adult sexuality. (http://www.sexualityandaging.com/)

More than Skin Deep: A Documentary About Self-Esteem (2001). Brooklyn and Toronto: Fanlight Productions. This 25-minute documentary explores the importance of the beauty salon to women living in a nursing home. The film shares the stories of six residents and makes the connection between living well, aging with dignity, and looking good. (http://www.fanlight.com/catalog/films/363_mtsd.php)

Promoting Excellent Alternatives in Kansas Nursing Homes (PEAK). These training materials were developed by the Center on Aging at Kansas State University to teach nursing homes about person-centered care. One of the modules is specific to sexuality. (http://www.aging kansas.org/LongTermCare/PEAK/peak.htm#modules)

Sexuality Information and Education Council of the United States (SIECUS). This is a national nonprofit organization that affirms sexuality as a natural and healthy part of living. (http://www.siecus.org)

Chapter 2. Sexuality and the Long-Term Care Resident

Back Seat Bingo. This short, animated video is about romance in older adulthood. The Center on Aging at Kansas State University uses this film to help viewers see sexuality as a normal part of aging. It can be purchased at this website: http://www.filmmovement.com/filmcatalog/index.asp?MerchandiseID=98.

Still Doing It. Harriman, NY: New Day Films. Nine women share honestly and with humor how they feel about themselves, sex, and love in later life. (http://www.newday.com/films/StillDoingIt.html)

Butler, R. (2002). *The New Love and Sex after 60.* New York: Ballantine Books. Try any of Butler's books, but this one is a classic. When it was first introduced in 1976, a Florida newspaper refused to advertise it because they thought it was too racy.

Ingersoll, T. S., & Scott, S. (n.d.). Sexuality policy guidelines for a geriatric residential facility. This document provides guidance for the construction of a sexuality policy. The authors use research literature to make a case for sexuality in long-term care. Retrieved from http://www. scribd.com/doc/18551910/Sample-Geriatric-Residence-Sexuality-Policy.

Index

Note: *f* indicates figures, *t* indicates tables, *sb* indicates sidebars, and *a* indicates activities.

Abuse
  case studies, 86–87
  dementia and, 111*sb*, 112
  of LGBT residents, 164
  sexual, 54–55, 139*sb*, 146, 147*sb*, 148
  by staff, 148–149
Acceptance, 16, 83–84, 89
Acquired immunodeficiency syndrome (AIDS),
      see HIV/AIDS
Activities
  dementia, 123–133
  environment and privacy, 207–212
  family influences, 71–72, 91–98
  health and sexuality, 225–226
  inappropriate behavior, 151–153
  LGBT residents, 169–182
  long-term care residents, 31–41
  policy, 209–211, 243–249
  sexuality framework, 11
  staff attitudes on sexuality, 65–76
AD, *see* Alzheimer's disease
ADA, *see* Americans with Disabilities Act
ADA Accessibility Guidelines (ADAAG), 193
ADAAG, *see* ADA Accessibility Guidelines
      (ADAAG)
Administration, 51, 61
Admissions process
  gender neutral language and, 165–166
  policy and, 234, 238, 241*sb*
  sexual history taking in, 142–144, 234
  sexual orientation questions in, 163*sb*
Adult children
  activities on, 71–72*a*
  ageism of, 44, 45*sb*
  as barriers to sexuality, 22
  parenting parents, 80
  paternal attitudes of, 88
  resident relationships and, 229
  see also Family influences
Adultery, 113–114, 115
  see also Extramarital relationships
Advocates
  ombudsmen, 7, 55, 227–228
  staff as, 27
Affection
  dementia and, 102–103, 104, 120
  move to long-term care and, 85, 104
  ways of showing, 20, 21*sb*

Age discrimination, *see* Ageism
Age Norms, 35–36*a*
Ageism
  activities on, 37*a*
  of adult children, 44, 45*sb*
  inappropriate behavior and, 140
  LGBT residents and, 156, 157, 162
  sexuality and, 19–20
  social age and, 254
Aggressiveness, sexual, 137–138, 141
Aging sexuality, 2
Aging stereotype(s), 19–20, 31–37, 158
Aging Stereotype Quiz, 31*a*, 33*a*
AIDS, *see* HIV/AIDS
Allen, Woody, 5*sb*
ALS (amyatrophic lateral sclerosis), 25
Alzheimer's disease (AD)
  assumptions on, 120–121
  case studies, 115, 251
  inappropriate behavior and, 141, 145*sb*
  intimacy seeking and, 140
  mental status and, 106–107*sb*
  overview of, 100, 101*t*
  sexual life of couples and, 103–104
  see also Dementia
Americans with Disabilities Act (ADA),
      192–193
Amyatrophic lateral sclerosis (ALS), 25
Anger, 82, 84
Assessment
  for consent, 104–113, 106–107*sb*, 108*sb*,
      110*sb*, 111*sb*
  of inappropriate behavior, 140–141, 215
  of LGBT inclusion, 179–182
  of sexual health, 215–216, 216*sb*
  for sexually transmitted diseases, 216*sb*, 220
Assisted living
  case studies, 148, 151, 251
  definition of, 7
  policy and, 232
Attention, 106–107*sb*, 120
Attitudes
  on condom purchases, 62
  of family, 78, 79*f*, 79*sb*, 87–89, 91, 97–98
  on lesbianism, 23*sb*
  on older lovers in films, 5*sb*
  of residents, 8, 14–19, 14*sb*, 15*t*, 16*f*, 20, 21*sb*, 22
  of staff, *see* Staff attitudes on sexuality